100 Questions & Answers About Menopause

by Rebecca Levy-Gantt, DO

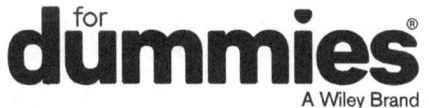

100 Questions & Answers About Menopause For Dummies®

Published by: **John Wiley & Sons, Inc.**, 111 River Street, Hoboken, NJ 07030-5774,
www.wiley.com

For general information on our other products and services, please contact our Customer
Care Department within the U.S. at 877-762-2974, outside the U.S. at 317-572-3993,
or fax 317-572-4002. For technical support, please visit https://hub.wiley.com/
community/support/dummies.

Wiley publishes in a variety of print and electronic formats and by print-on-demand.
Some material included with standard print versions of this book may not be included in
e-books or in print-on-demand. If this book refers to media that is not included in the
version you purchased, you may download this material at http://booksupport.wiley.
com. For more information about Wiley products, visit www.wiley.com.

Library of Congress Control Number is available from the publisher.

ISBN 978-1-394-36969-0 (pbk); ISBN 978-1-394-36971-3 (ebk);
ISBN 978-1-394-36970-6 (ebk)

Printed and bound by CPI Group (UK) Ltd, Croydon, CR0 4YY

C9781394369690_190126

Contents at a Glance

Introduction 1

Part 1: Understanding Menopause 3
CHAPTER 1: Introducing Menopause 5
CHAPTER 2: Heat, Sleep, and Mood 9

Part 2: Managing Menopause: Medication,
Lifestyle, and Alternative Therapies 15
CHAPTER 3: Medical Treatments and Therapies 17
CHAPTER 4: Making Lifestyle Changes 29
CHAPTER 5: Alternative Therapies 37

Part 3: Physical Health in Menopause 45
CHAPTER 6: Sexual, Reproductive, and Urinary Health 47
CHAPTER 7: Metabolism and the Endocrine System 61
CHAPTER 8: Cardiovascular Health 69
CHAPTER 9: Systemic Health 73
CHAPTER 10: Bones, Muscles, and Joints 85
CHAPTER 11: Skin, Hair, and Nails 91

Part 4: Cognitive and Emotional Health
in Menopause 101
CHAPTER 12: Cognitive and Sensory Health 103
CHAPTER 13: Mental and Emotional Health 113

Index 123

Table of Contents

INTRODUCTION 1

    About This Book 1

    Foolish Assumptions.. 2

    Icon Used in This Book 2

    Where to Go from Here... 2

PART 1: UNDERSTANDING MENOPAUSE.......................... 3

CHAPTER 1: **Introducing Menopause** 5

    What Is Menopause and When Does
It Usually Occur?.. 5

    What Is Perimenopause and How Is It
Different from Menopause? 6

    What Are the Most Common Symptoms
of Menopause?... 6

    How Long Do Menopausal Symptoms Last? 7

    How Can I Talk to My Doctor about
Menopausal Symptoms?... 7

    What Are the Long-Term Health Implications
of Menopause?... 8

CHAPTER 2: **Heat, Sleep, and Mood** 9

    What Are Hot Flashes?... 9

    What Are Night Sweats? 10

    Why Does Menopause Cause Changes
in Body Temperature Regulation? 10

    How Does Menopause Affect Sleep? 11

    Is Estrogen the Only Option for Regulating
Hot Flashes, Night Sweats, and Sleep
Disturbances?... 12

    What Are the Psychological Effects
of Menopause?... 13

    How Can Psychological Issues Related
to Menopause Be Treated?..................................... 13

PART 2: MANAGING MENOPAUSE: MEDICATION, LIFESTYLE, AND ALTERNATIVE THERAPIES......................15

CHAPTER 3: **Medical Treatments and Therapies**...............17

What Kind of Hormones Are Available
to Take in Menopause? 18

Who Cannot Take Hormones in Menopause?.......19

What Are the Benefits of Taking Birth
Control Pills during Menopause? 21

What Are the Risks of Taking Birth
Control Pills during Menopause? 22

Should Women Take Testosterone
in Menopause? 23

Are There Other Prescription Medications
That Can Be Used for Hot Flashes?.......................24

How Do I Treat My Menopausal Symptoms
If I've Had Breast Cancer?..25

How Do I Treat My Menopausal Symptoms
If I've Had Ovarian or Endometrial Cancer?..........26

CHAPTER 4: **Making Lifestyle Changes**...............................29

What Are the Benefits of Lifestyle Changes
for Menopause Symptoms?....................................30

Can Dietary Changes Help with Menopause
Symptoms? 31

What Are the Benefits of Nutritional
Counseling for Menopausal Symptoms? 33

Are There Any Foods I Should Avoid during
Menopause? 34

What Role Does Exercise Play in Managing
Menopausal Symptoms?...34

Can Menopause Cause Weight Gain?....................35

What Are the Best Ways to Manage
Weight during Menopause?....................................36

CHAPTER 5: **Alternative Therapies**....................................37

What Are the Benefits of Mindfulness
and Meditation during Menopause? 38

What Are the Benefits of Acupuncture
during Menopause?...38

What Are the Benefits of Yoga in Menopause?.....39

What Are the Benefits of Aromatherapy
for Relieving Menopausal Symptoms? 40

What Are the Benefits of Massage Therapy
for Menopausal Symptoms?....................................41

What Are the Benefits of Chiropractic Care
for Menopause? 42

What Are the Benefits of Herbal Remedies
for Menopausal Symptoms?....................................43

PART 3: PHYSICAL HEALTH IN MENOPAUSE..................45

CHAPTER 6: **Sexual, Reproductive, and Urinary
Health** 47

How Does Menopause Affect Relationships
and Intimacy?..48

How Does Menopause Affect Sexual Health?........48

How Does Menopause Affect Libido?.....................49

How Can I Increase My Libido If It's
Disappearing?..50

Can Menopause Cause Vaginal Dryness
and Discomfort?..52

What Is Available for Vaginal Dryness
in Menopause? 53

How Do Hormones Impact Genital Tissues? 55

How Does Menopause Affect Reproductive
Organs? 56

How Does Menopause Affect Reproductive
Cycles? 57

How Does Menopause Impact Reproductive
Hormones?...57

How Does Menopause Impact Urinary Health? 58

Do I Still Need a Pap Smear in Menopause?..........59

CHAPTER 7: **Metabolism and the Endocrine System** 61

How Does Menopause Affect Metabolic
Health?..62

Can Menopause Cause Changes in Blood
Sugar Levels? 62

Can Menopause Increase Risk for Diabetes? 63

Can Menopause Cause Changes in Appetite?.......64

How Does Menopause Affect the Endocrine
System? 65

How Does Menopause Affect Thyroid Health?......66

How Does Menopause Impact Adrenal Health?......66

How Does Menopause Cause Changes
in the Cholesterol Profile?...............................67

What Affect Does Menopause Have
on Bone-Regulating Hormones? 68

CHAPTER 8: **Cardiovascular Health**..69

How Does Menopause Affect Cardiovascular
Health?..70

How Can I Maintain Heart Health during
Menopause? 70

How Does Menopause Impact Cholesterol
Levels? 71

Can Menopause Cause Changes in Blood
Pressure?..72

CHAPTER 9: **Systemic Health**..73

Can Menopause Increase the Risk of
Certain Cancers? 73

How Does Menopause Affect Gastrointestinal
Health?..75

What Are Some Common Gastrointestinal
Symptoms Associated with Menopause?..............75

How Does Menopause Affect Respiratory
Health?..76

How Does Menopause Impact Liver Health?.........77

How Does Menopause Affect Kidney Health? 78

How Does Menopause Affect Oral Health? 78

Can Menopause Cause Changes in Body Odor?.....79

How Does Menopause Affect the
Immune System?..80

What Are the Best Ways to Manage
Menopause-Related Fatigue? 81

How Does Menopause Affect Musculoskeletal
Health?..82

How Can I Best Treat Balance Problems
in Menopause? 83

CHAPTER 10: **Bones, Muscles, and Joints** 85

How Much Does Menopause Affect Bone
Health?..85

Can Menopause Cause Joint Pain and Stiffness?.....86

Can Menopause Cause Changes in Muscle
Mass and Strength? 86

Can I Take Supplements to Help Build New
Muscle?..88

What Kind of Supplements Can Help
Menopausal Bones?..89

CHAPTER 11: **Skin, Hair, and Nails**................................91

How Does Menopause Impact Skin? 91

How Does Menopause Affect Hair? 92

How Can I Best Take Care of Menopausal Skin?......93

How Can Menopause Cause Changes
in Skin Pigmentation? 94

What Are the Best Ways to Manage
Menopausal Hair Loss? 95

Can Menopause Cause Changes in Nail
Health?..96

What Lifestyle Strategies Can Help
Menopausal Skin, Hair, and Nails?..........................97

Why Might Menopausal Women Find
an Increase in Facial or Body Hair but
Thinner Scalp Hair?..98

PART 4: COGNITIVE AND EMOTIONAL HEALTH IN MENOPAUSE..101

CHAPTER 12: **Cognitive and Sensory Health**........................103

Can Menopause Cause Memory Problems
or Cognitive Changes?..104

What Can I Do to Improve Cognitive
Function in Menopause?......................................105

What Is the Connection between
Menopause and Dementia?..................................106

Can Menopause Cause Changes
in Vision and Eye Health?....................................108

Can Menopause Cause Changes
in Taste and Smell?..108

Can Menopause Cause Changes in Hearing?........109

What Kind of Neurological Symptoms
Can Occur in Menopause?...................................109

How Does Menopause Affect the Body's
Circadian Rhythm?..110

CHAPTER 13: **Mental and Emotional Health**........................113

What Are the Best Ways to Manage
Menopause-Related Anxiety?...............................114

What Are the Best Ways to Manage
Menopause-Related Depression?..........................115

What Are the Best Ways to Manage
Menopause-Related Irritability?...........................117

What Are the Best Ways to Manage
Menopause-Related Mood Swings?........................118

What Are Some Effective Ways to
Manage Stress during Menopause?.......................119

What Are the Benefits of Cognitive
Behavioral Therapy for Menopausal
Symptoms?...120

Are There Support Groups for Women
Going through Menopause?.................................121

INDEX...123

Introduction

According to the World Health Organization, more than one-quarter of the world's population are women age 50 or older, and those women are, or soon will be, menopausal. Yet many women approach or experience menopause knowing very little about it. I wrote this book to answer common questions about menopause — what it is, how menopause affects the body and mind, and the treatment options available for troublesome symptoms.

About This Book

This book is a reference, which means you don't need to read the chapters in order from beginning to end and you don't have to remember anything — there isn't a test at the end of it.

Within this book, you may note that some web addresses break across two lines of text. If you're reading this book in print and want to visit one of these web pages, simply key in the web address exactly as it's noted in the text, pretending as though the line break doesn't exist. If you're reading this as an e-book, you've got it easy — just click the web address to be taken directly to the web page.

Foolish Assumptions

In writing this book, I made just a couple of assumptions about you, the reader:

» You're approaching menopause or are already in menopause.

» You have questions, and you want answers.

If those basic assumptions apply to you, you've come to the right place.

Icon Used in This Book

This book uses the following icon in the margins:

TIP

When you see the Tip icon, you'll find information that will make your life a little easier, at least when it comes to menopause.

Where to Go from Here

If you aren't sure where to begin, head to the Table of Contents and skim through the questions until you find one that catches your eye. Or, if you have a specific topic in mind, search for it in the Index. Want to know absolutely everything? Turn the page and start with Part 1.

1

Understanding Menopause

IN THIS PART . . .

This part explains what menopause is, when it happens, and the common symptoms many people experience — from hot flashes to trouble sleeping to mood swings. If you want the basics on menopause, this part is for you.

Chapter **1**

Introducing Menopause

E very woman who lives long enough will go through menopause. By definition, menopause is the time in a woman's life when the ovaries stop functioning. In this chapter, I explain what menopause and perimenopause are, the common symptoms of menopause, and some of the long-term health implications of menopause.

What Is Menopause and When Does It Usually Occur?

Menopause is defined by the time in a woman's life where the possibility of natural reproduction ends. The ovaries are no longer making hormones (estrogen, progesterone, and testosterone), and ovulation is no longer occurring. Menstruation ceases, and when 12 months have passed with no periods, a woman is officially in menopause. In the United States, the average age of menopause is 51.

What Is Perimenopause and How Is It Different from Menopause?

Perimenopause is the approximately four to seven years leading up to menopause. A hallmark of perimenopause is that menstrual periods usually begin to come with some irregularity. Periods may be more than once in a month or skip months altogether; they may become heavier or lighter, or change to a different pattern than previously seen. When 12 period-free months have passed, that marks the arrival of menopause.

What Are the Most Common Symptoms of Menopause?

The most common symptoms of menopause are hot flashes, night sweats, vaginal dryness, brain fog, poor concentration, weight gain, low energy, lack of libido, insomnia, mood swings, and changes in bladder function. Most women do not have all of these symptoms, but many women have at least some of them.

How Long Do Menopausal Symptoms Last?

Menopausal symptoms can last anywhere from one to ten years — quite a range. The average amount of time is four to ten years. Symptoms often start before the end of menstrual periods. The severity of symptoms can wax and wane for years. The symptom of vaginal dryness is likely to be ongoing unless some type of treatment is initiated.

How Can I Talk to My Doctor about Menopausal Symptoms?

The best way to discuss menopausal symptoms is to start by finding a doctor who specializes in menopause. Sometimes a trusted friend will have seen a physician they would recommend, or check online at https://menopause.org for a practitioner near your location. Then make a separate appointment just to discuss menopausal symptoms and to make a plan. (Don't try to bring up all menopausal issues at an annual physical or at a visit where you're having a procedure done — there won't be enough time to discuss it all.)

At this special consultation visit, bring a list of very specific questions that you'd like the doctor to answer for you, and list them in order of importance. If you don't get to discuss all your questions in the first visit, you can schedule another visit to make sure you get all your questions answered — but at least you'll get your most pressing questions answered first, and you can see if that practitioner is a good fit.

What Are the Long-Term Health Implications of Menopause?

Menopausal symptoms that are not relieved — like severe hot flashes and night sweats — can be red flags for future cardiovascular illness. When there are ongoing hot flashes, it's a sign of inflamed blood vessels and possible vascular disease, which can cause medical problems over time. When night sweats cause frequent waking and don't allow for long stretches of deep rapid eye movement (REM) sleep, it can often result in metabolic disease, weight gain, low energy, fatigue, and a lack of focus and concentration. Physical symptoms that are not treated — like vaginal dryness — can ultimately result in urinary tract problems and thinning vaginal tissues, leading to pain and difficulty with sexual activity.

Chapter **2**

Heat, Sleep, and Mood

Menopause can bring a whole host of changes to your body and mind — some temporary, others not — but the three most common are hot flashes, night sweats, and trouble sleeping. The good news is that all three of these symptoms can be treated successfully — you don't have to suffer through them. This chapter covers all three of the most common symptoms and offers tips on how to manage them.

What Are Hot Flashes?

Hot flashes are a sensation of overwhelming warmth that occurs throughout the body periodically (and sometimes randomly). These flashes can be felt as a sensation of heat rising from the trunk up through the chest, neck, and most notably, in the face. Skin can get clammy, and the flash is usually followed by sweating.

TIP

You can manage hot flashes by using fans, wearing lighter clothes, or taking various medications designed to control them.

What Are Night Sweats?

Night sweats are one of the most common and disruptive symptoms of menopause, causing poor sleep, fatigue, and low energy. Night sweats generally follow a particular pattern: As you sleep, the temperature regulation area of the brain somehow senses that your body is too hot and needs to release the heat; this causes sweating, and as the sweat evaporates from the skin, you wake up, feel sweaty and chilly, and then typically need to change clothes and sometimes even bedsheets in order to go back to sleep.

Why Does Menopause Cause Changes in Body Temperature Regulation?

Estrogen plays a key role in regulating body temperature, and the decline in estrogen disrupts this regulation. Estrogen acts on an area of the brain called the *hypothalamus.* This part of the brain helps maintain a zone of comfortable body temperature. When estrogen declines, the hypothalamus becomes more sensitive to minor changes in body temperature, and the balance is disrupted. This leads to hot flashes and night sweats, which are hallmarks of menopause.

How Does Menopause Affect Sleep?

Sleep patterns become disrupted for various reasons during menopause. The most common type of disrupted sleep occurs from night sweats. If sweating during the night causes you to wake up, treating the sweating will help provide relief.

You may also have trouble falling asleep or staying asleep, separate from night sweats. Estrogen and progesterone usually have a calming effect, promoting sleep. When your levels of estrogen and progesterone drop (as they do during menopause), falling asleep and staying asleep may be more difficult.

Other causes for sleep disturbances can include increased inflammation and muscle pain, as well as frequent urination, all of which can occur as estrogen levels drop.

Is Estrogen the Only Option for Regulating Hot Flashes, Night Sweats, and Sleep Disturbances?

TIP

Taking estrogen can help regulate symptoms having to do with body temperature regulation, such as hot flashes and night sweats. But newer medications are available for menopause, too. These newer options work directly on the hypothalamus (the part of the brain that helps maintain a comfortable body temperature) to relieve hot flashes, bypassing the need for estrogen. They work very well in women who can't or don't want to use estrogen.

If other symptoms are disrupting sleep, getting to the root cause of the disruptions may help. Sleep that is disturbed by muscle or joint pain may be relieved by a bedtime routine involving gentle stretching, moist heat, or anti-inflammatory medications. Women with irritable bladder symptoms causing the need to urinate frequently may be awakened in the middle of the night; limiting fluids, caffeine, or alcohol close to bedtime may help, and medications to treat overactive bladder can be used in the right circumstances as well.

TIP

Addressing poor sleep in menopause is extremely important for maintaining good health and cognitive function.

What Are the Psychological Effects of Menopause?

The menopause years often coincide with other concerns that women have about aging in general — for example, worries about declining health, body changes, relationship shifts, aging parents, and children leaving home. All these issues may be part of the identity transformation that can take place around this time. Many women face new or heightened anxieties about these changes, making some of them more irritable, tearful, or sensitive. Hormonal changes may play a role, making mood shifts more likely, but for many women these psychological effects are temporary.

How Can Psychological Issues Related to Menopause Be Treated?

Sometimes anxiety and depression present during the transition to menopause, but those most at risk are women who had these conditions in their younger years, especially at times of other transitions (puberty, pregnancy, postpartum).

Hormones may play a role in new-onset psychological symptoms, but these symptoms must be evaluated on a case-by-case basis and not just assumed to be from shifting or transitioning hormones, in order to be properly assessed and treated.

For many women, successful treatment will combine a hormonal solution along with those that address anxiety, depression, and other mood disorders.

If mood changes are partially triggered by poor sleep or hot flashes, they can be remedied by good sleep hygiene and treatment geared toward relieving the hot flashes.

TIP

2

Managing Menopause: Medication, Lifestyle, and Alternative Therapies

This part outlines the medical treatments available to treat the symptoms of menopause — from menopausal hormone therapy (MHT) to nonhormonal options. It also covers lifestyle changes you can make to manage symptoms, including modifying your diet and exercise routine. Finally, this part explores alternative therapies for managing the symptoms of menopause — including meditation, yoga, acupuncture, massage, and more.

Chapter **3**

Medical Treatments and Therapies

I f your menopausal symptoms are bothering you, you may be interested in prescription medication, including menopausal hormone therapy. Or you may be unable to take hormones and be curious what else is available. This chapter talks about all things medication — what options are available, who can (and can't) take them, and what symptoms they may relieve.

What Kind of Hormones Are Available to Take in Menopause?

The term *menopausal hormone therapy* usually refers to the use of one or more of the following:

» **Estrogen** (usually in the form of estradiol, which is the body's most abundant form of estrogen)

» **Progesterone** (or something called a progestin, which is similar to progesterone)

» Possibly **testosterone**

Estrogen comes in many different forms: oral pills, patches, gels, lotions, sprays, and a vaginal ring. One type of vaginal ring provides only local treatment to the vaginal tissues; another type of ring, at a higher dose, acts on the body as an estrogen pill, patch, or cream would, relieving systemic symptoms.

One of the rules of prescribing estrogen therapy in menopause is that if a woman still has her uterus, she should also take progesterone or some form of progestin. Estrogen — whether in a pill, patch, gel, or the higher-dose vaginal ring — can cause blood and tissue to build up inside the uterus, so taking progesterone or progestin acts as a safeguard, not allowing the blood and lining to build up too much.

Estrogen and progesterone relieve many menopausal symptoms like hot flashes, night sweats, insomnia, low energy, and more. Estrogen can help prevent bones from thinning, and progesterone may also act as a mood stabilizer.

Testosterone levels drop in menopause as well (although some studies have shown that testosterone levels may rise again somewhat in women in their 60s). The one menopausal symptom that is an indication for adding testosterone into the menopause hormone plan is lack of interest in sex, in which the lack of interest is not related to relationship problems, medical conditions, depression, or another treatable condition.

TIP

A physician or practitioner who is familiar with hormones and menopause should help decide which combination and which doses of menopausal hormones are effective and safe for your individual treatment plan. It may take a few different combinations to arrive at the plan that provides the most relief for you.

Who Cannot Take Hormones in Menopause?

Although menopausal hormone therapy can be very effective at managing menopausal symptoms, it isn't recommended or safe for everyone. Women who fall into the following categories should not take hormones in menopause:

> » Women with a history of breast cancer, especially cancer that is *estrogen positive* (meaning that the cancer can respond to

and be stimulated by estrogen): There may be some exceptions depending on the type and stage of the cancer, but that requires evaluation and discussion with a physician familiar with the specifics and history of that particular cancer.

» **Women who were thought to be menopausal (no period for 12 months) and then have unexpected bleeding:** These women are not candidates for menopausal hormone therapy until and unless that bleeding is evaluated. Unexplained bleeding can be caused by cancer, so that must be ruled out prior to using hormones.

» **Women with a history of a stroke, heart attack, or blood clot (also called *deep vein thrombosis*):** These women are generally not thought to be candidates for hormone therapy, because estrogen can increase the risk of a recurrence. (Depending on the individual situation, they *may* be able to use estrogen that is delivered through the skin.)

» **Women over the age of 60 who smoke.**

» **Women with active liver disease.**

» **Women with uncontrolled high blood pressure:** If the blood pressure is controlled, even with medication, these women may be candidates for certain types of hormone therapy.

There are some conditions that may not be absolute reasons that a woman can't use hormone therapy, but these conditions require further thought and possible investigation before a hormone plan can be safely implemented, and the risks and benefits should be discussed. These conditions include:

» Active gallbladder disease
» Extremely high triglycerides
» Borderline blood pressure
» Mild cardiac disease

Initiation of any hormone therapy plan should always include a discussion of medical history, looking for possible reasons that the hormones may worsen current medical conditions or cause harm.

What Are the Benefits of Taking Birth Control Pills during Menopause?

Because menopause, by definition, is a time in which ovarian function ceases, and one of the functions of the ovaries is to produce eggs (or *ovulate*), there is rarely if ever, a need for birth control pills during menopause. Without ovulation, there can be no pregnancy, and because birth control pills are designed to prevent pregnancy, they're unnecessary in menopause.

However, birth control pills are often used for other reasons:

» To control heavy bleeding (which should not be something occurring in menopause)

» For mood stability (which *may* be a reason to use a birth control pill in early menopause or in the transition to menopause)

» To treat hot flashes

TIP

Birth control pills contain hormones in much higher doses than the doses typically used in menopausal hormone therapy plans, and rarely are these higher doses required to provide symptom relief in menopause.

What Are the Risks of Taking Birth Control Pills during Menopause?

Oral birth control pills carry a higher risk of blood clots and stroke than menopausal hormones (especially if those menopausal hormones go through the skin like a patch or a cream). Menopausal symptoms like hot flashes or night sweats can usually easily be treated with the lower doses in typical menopausal hormone plans.

Also, when women are of menopausal age, risk for other medical conditions (including high blood pressure, heart disease, and high cholesterol) is higher, and the combination of oral birth control pills along with these medical conditions increases the risk of heart attack, stroke, and blood clots.

TIP

Menopausal hormonal treatment is designed to relieve symptoms and lower risk. This can usually be done without using the doses found in a birth control pill.

Should Women Take Testosterone in Menopause?

Currently the only indication for prescribing testosterone for women in menopause that has research and evidence behind it is for low libido, after evaluation by a medical practitioner trained in menopausal hormone management. In the United States, the Food and Drug Administration (FDA) has not approved any type of testosterone for women. The same applies in most other countries — however, Australia, New Zealand, South Africa, and the United Kingdom have an approved testosterone product, and many countries allow off-label use of testosterone for women, in doses much lower than the doses used for men.

There is some evidence that taking or using testosterone may have a positive impact on low libido in women. Many women also report relief from joint pain, muscle aches, and inflammation, as well as an increase in energy, but these are all anecdotal reports and not specific indications for prescribing testosterone.

Well-known side effects of taking too much testosterone can include acne, oily skin, changes in liver function and cholesterol, and deepening of the voice. However, these side effects do not usually occur at the safe doses used for the treatment of low libido. If your doctor prescribes testosterone, they should check your blood levels of testosterone to be sure the dose isn't too high.

Are There Other Prescription Medications That Can Be Used for Hot Flashes?

Currently several nonhormonal prescription medications are approved to treat hot flashes:

» **Fezolinetant and elinzanetant:** These two are the most recently approved. They're in a category called *neurokinin receptor antagonists,* because they work on the center of the brain that regulates body temperature. They're both once-a-day oral medications designed to treat hot flashes and night sweats, and they're very effective. They do have some potential side effects (including nausea, diarrhea, and rarely, a possible effect on liver function).

» **Gabapentin:** A medication originally prescribed for seizures or nerve pain, gabapentin can also treat hot flashes. It's usually taken two to three times a day, and it may have some side effects like dizziness or sleepiness.

» **Oxybutynin:** A medication originally prescribed for overactive bladder symptoms, oxybutynin is also effective for relieving hot flashes. It may have a side effect of dry mouth, and there is some indication that if it's used for a long period of time, it may have a detrimental effect on cognitive function.

» **Paroxetine:** Paroxetine is an antidepressant and antianxiety medication at a 10- or 20-milligram dose. It's approved for the treatment of hot flashes at the dose of 7.5 milligrams per day. It may cause some side effects (like nausea and headaches).

How Do I Treat My Menopausal Symptoms If I've Had Breast Cancer?

In general, women who have had breast cancer are usually not candidates for hormone therapy. In certain circumstances, depending on the type of cancer, there may be some hormones that can be part of a menopause treatment plan. If you've had breast cancer, you should talk with a physician about whether you may safely use hormones and what your individual risks may be.

TIP
There are many alternatives to hormones that may be used to relieve menopausal symptoms (see the preceding section).

Non-medication methods to relieve menopausal symptoms include cognitive behavioral therapy (CBT) and eliminating triggers like caffeine and alcohol. Some women use supplements to relieve hot flashes, but there are no robust studies to prove that they work.

One symptom that most experts agree on treating is vaginal dryness. Even women who have had breast cancer can usually use low-dose topical vaginal estrogen if other nonhormonal methods seem to bring relief.

TIP
Talk with your physician before using any treatment to manage menopausal symptoms after a breast cancer diagnosis.

How Do I Treat My Menopausal Symptoms If I've Had Ovarian or Endometrial Cancer?

Most women who have been diagnosed with ovarian cancer or endometrial cancer (also known as uterine cancer) have had surgery, usually including a *hysterectomy* (removal of the uterus) and *oophorectomy* (removal of the ovaries).

Details of the specific type of cancer and what type of cancer treatment has been done should be reviewed by a physician to determine whether hormonal treatments would be safe or recommended. Some types of ovarian cancers and most types of endometrial cancers can be stimulated by estrogen, so even after removal of the uterus and/or ovaries, it may not be recommended to use estrogen in these cases.

TIP

Vaginal symptoms like dryness can usually be treated after surgery with hormonal or nonhormonal methods, even with a history of ovarian or endometrial cancer. Women having hot flashes and night sweats can usually take nonhormonal medications regardless of cancer history.

Chapter **4**

Making Lifestyle Changes

Although medications are available to treat the symptoms of menopause (see Chapter 3), you may not need them. Whether your symptoms are minor or you just aren't interested in taking medication, some simple lifestyle modifications can make a big difference. This chapter covers everything from diet and exercise to stress management.

What Are the Benefits of Lifestyle Changes for Menopause Symptoms?

Menopause is a great time to reevaluate lifestyle habits that may or may not be working. Not everyone needs a complete overhaul of their daily routine — even small changes can help manage the enormous physical, mental, and psychological changes that take place starting in the perimenopause years and continuing on through menopause. Being intentional with lifestyle plans and decisions can make the transition to menopause and the future years more manageable, empowering, and positive.

Here are some lifestyle changes and how they can improve the symptoms of menopause:

» **Being more active:** Even if you've never been active before, it's essential to be active in menopause. Combining strength training (for example, using light weights, elastic bands, or body weight as resistance) with cardiovascular activity (such as hiking, walking, running, swimming, or aerobic classes) will preserve muscle and bone function and heart health and help you maintain a healthy weight. Balance training and stretching can help lower inflammation and decrease the risk of falls and fractures, too.

» **Getting enough sleep:** Sleep *must* be a priority. Poor sleep should be evaluated to get to the root of the problem, whether it's from hormonal disruptions, sleep apnea, irregular bedtime habits, or a medical condition. Sleep deprivation worsens any ongoing medical problems and will intensify menopausal symptoms.

» **Managing stress:** Menopause can be a time of stress, and you can manage or lessen it in many ways. Yoga, meditation, counseling, CBT, and exercise are just a few ways to deal with stressors that can occur or worsen in the menopause years.

» **Eating healthily and intentionally:** Include the important foods in the diet like high-quality plant protein, and avoid processed foods and alcohol.

TIP

It's never too late to adopt healthy lifestyle habits. There is plenty of evidence that the basis for feeling better in menopause and relieving symptoms starts with a healthy lifestyle.

Can Dietary Changes Help with Menopause Symptoms?

There is no special diet recommended in menopause, but incorporating fruits, vegetables, lean proteins, nuts, and seeds into your diet, while limiting or eliminating the intake of excess sugar, saturated fats, and highly processed foods, is the basis of a healthy diet, in menopause or at any stage of life.

Several specific diets can incorporate these dietary components:

» **Dietary Approaches to Stop Hypertension (DASH)** emphasizes nutrient-rich foods, including fruits, vegetables, whole grains, lean proteins, low-fat dairy, nuts, seeds, and healthy fats. This diet can provide a well-balanced intake of needed nutrients.

» **The Mediterranean diet** is based on the traditional eating patterns of people who live in countries bordering the Mediterranean Sea. Its focus is on whole, nutrient-dense foods; healthy fats; and a balance of plant-based and lean, animal-based ingredients.

» **The plant-based diet** has an emphasis on vegetables; fruits; healthy, plant-based proteins like beans and tofu; nuts; and plant-based oils.

TIP

No matter which diet you follow, it should include a variety of nutritious foods for overall health, maintain heart and brain function, and provide energy for daily activities. Most of all, it should be healthy, enjoyable, and sustainable for a lifetime.

What Are the Benefits of Nutritional Counseling for Menopausal Symptoms?

A nutritional counselor will discuss what you should include in your diet:

» **High-quality protein:** Protein combats the decline in muscle mass that may naturally occur during menopause. Some high-protein foods are eggs, chicken, turkey, fish, tofu, lentils, Greek yogurt, legumes, nuts, and seeds.

» **Foods with calcium:** Calcium is helpful in maintaining strong bones and decreasing the risk of osteoporosis and fractures. Examples of calcium-rich foods include fortified plant milks, dairy, leafy green vegetables, and sardines with bones.

» **Foods with omega-3 fatty acids:** Omega-3 fatty acids can support heart health and reduce inflammation. You can get omega-3 fatty acids in fatty fish (like salmon, sardines, and mackerel), seeds (like chia seeds and flaxseeds), and walnuts.

» **Fiber:** Fiber helps maintain gastrointestinal health and supports regular daily bowel movements. You can get it from vegetables and fruits with the skins on, whole grains like oats and quinoa, beans, and seeds.

TIP

A nutritional counselor can be helpful, but if you can't visit a nutritional counselor, you can read about specific eating plans on your own. The Academy of Nutrition and Dietetics has nutrition information at www.eatright.org/nutrition, and the Menopause Network has all kinds of info at https://menopausenetwork.org.

Are There Any Foods I Should Avoid during Menopause?

Just as there are foods to include in the diet during menopause, there are some foods to limit or avoid altogether.

Ultra-processed foods — like prepackaged and microwavable snacks and sugary foods, cereals, fast foods, and processed meats — can worsen inflammation, cause increased blood sugar (increasing the risk of prediabetes and diabetes), and contribute to poor sleep and fatigue.

Also, limit or eliminate alcohol altogether — it's high in sugar and can worsen hot flashes and insomnia. Not a good combination.

What Role Does Exercise Play in Managing Menopausal Symptoms?

Regular exercise in menopause can improve mood, sleep, and mental health. Exercise releases natural mood boosters called *endorphins,* which can improve sleep quality and reduce depression and anxiety. Gentle mobility exercises and low-impact workouts like swimming or yoga can help decrease inflammation and reduce stiffness.

Cardiovascular exercise has been shown to help relieve menopausal symptoms like hot flashes. This type of exercise is anything that elevates the heart rate and makes you sweat. Think: jogging, walking, hiking, biking, swimming, or aerobic classes. Aim for 30 to 45 minutes at a time, four to six times per week.

Weight-bearing activity (any exercise done while standing) and resistance exercises (with handheld weights or weight machines) can help keep your bones strong.

Balance and stretching exercises can help reduce the risk of falls.

TIP

Active Menopause Life (www.activemenopause life.com) is a website focused specifically on fitness for women going through menopause.

Can Menopause Cause Weight Gain?

Menopause itself does not automatically result in weight gain. The combination of a decrease in hormones, poor sleep, life stressors, a more sedentary lifestyle, and poor dietary choices combine to cause an average weight gain of 2 to 3 pounds per year throughout the menopausal years.

TIP

You can combine changes in diet, exercise, sleep, and stress management to prevent menopausal weight gain, or at least keep it to a minimum.

What Are the Best Ways to Manage Weight during Menopause?

There is a lot of evidence that a diet rich in healthy plant-based proteins, fiber, and fruits and vegetables is the best type of diet to follow in perimenopause and menopause. Specific dietary patterns, like the Mediterranean diet or intermittent fasting, may also be successful ways to manage weight and minimize weight gain in menopause. Exercise — including cardiovascular exercise and resistance training — are important components of a healthy menopause plan as well.

Chapter **5**

Alternative Therapies

When you're going through menopause, you may find yourself bombarded with ads on social media for every possible alternative therapy under the sun, or a well-meaning friend or relative may suggest some supplement or other. Here's the truth: Many alternative therapies haven't been studied or proven effective, and though some probably won't hurt, some can be dangerous.

In this chapter, I explain which alternative therapies are effective for which symptoms, so you don't waste your time on approaches that don't work or may cause even bigger problems.

What Are the Benefits of Mindfulness and Meditation during Menopause?

You may be able to address the emotional and physical symptoms of menopause through mindfulness practice. Mindfulness techniques teach awareness of bodily sensations without judgment. They include deep breathing techniques, body scanning, yoga, and stress reduction, all of which can lead to better sleep and a reduction of the intensity of hot flashes and other menopausal symptoms.

Meditation works on the mind–body connection to help manage symptoms and relieve stress. It helps reduce the body's stress response, which may help lessen the intensity and frequency of hot flashes. Studies have shown that meditation can help cognition, improve sleep quality, and lessen depressive symptoms in menopause.

What Are the Benefits of Acupuncture during Menopause?

Several small studies have concluded that acupuncture may reduce hot flashes and night sweats in menopause. Menopausal women have also seen improvements in quality-of-life measures like sleep, memory, and cognitive symptoms and moods with the use of regular acupuncture treatments. Some studies have shown that when menopausal women use "usual measures" like hormones and other medications to reduce hot flashes, *adding* acupuncture to their treatment plan can provide further improvement of these symptoms. Some larger reviews of multiple studies found significant reductions in the frequency and severity of hot flashes while having acupuncture treatments, and those effects can last for three months after treatments cease.

What Are the Benefits of Yoga in Menopause?

Yoga that concentrates on relaxation, flexibility, balance, and weight-bearing poses can have numerous benefits at any age, especially in menopause. Yoga can help maintain bone density and muscle strength and reduce the risk of falls. Calming breath work can help improve sleep and relieve anxiety.

TIP

Specific yoga sequences can help with specific targets:

» **For relaxation and sleep,** seated breathing, legs-up-on-the-wall pose, and guided relaxation may help.

» **For strength and balance,** poses that focus on posture like the chair pose, bridge pose, and triangle pose may provide those benefits.

There is not much evidence for yoga as a way to relieve menopausal symptoms like hot flashes and night sweats, but some women report reduced frequency or intensity of those symptoms with regular practice of yoga.

You don't need to practice yoga at an in-person class; many good yoga apps and YouTube channels are available, including the following:

» **Yoga with Adriene:** Adriene Mishler is an Austin, Texas–based yoga instructor with a following of more than 13 million people on her wildly popular YouTube channel (www.youtube.com/yogawithadriene).

» **Yoga for Beginners:** This app has easy-to-follow sessions including chair yoga and meditation. Search Google Play or the Apple App Store to find the app for your device.

What Are the Benefits of Aromatherapy for Relieving Menopausal Symptoms?

Aromatherapy has been said to work by stimulating smell receptors via diffusion or through steam, with the goal of improving emotional, physical, or mental well-being. Evidence for aromatherapy is mostly anecdotal, but some people say that certain essential oils used in aromatherapy may confer some benefits in menopause. Lavender or chamomile scents may have a somewhat calming effect, promoting relaxation. They may also help with sleep, although research is often small scale and limited.

There is no evidence that aromatherapy helps with hot flashes or night sweats, the most common symptoms for which menopausal women seek relief.

TIP

Some oils may interact with medications or make certain conditions worse, including hormonal-mediated conditions, so talk with your healthcare practitioner before starting an aromatherapy plan.

What Are the Benefits of Massage Therapy for Menopausal Symptoms?

Often, women in menopause complain of achiness in their muscles, sore muscles and joints, anxiety, and difficulty sleeping. Massage therapy can address many of these symptoms in a supportive way. It can promote relaxation, making it easier to fall asleep and stay asleep; it can relieve aches and stiffness in joints and muscles. Often declining levels of estrogen are associated with joint pain and swelling and inflammation of muscles, and massage therapy can be a way to alleviate these symptoms. Massage can help improve circulation and reduce muscle stress.

Various types of massage are thought to have specific effects on the body. For example, Swedish massage may be better for relaxation, stress relief, and better sleep. Shiatsu massage focuses on particular acupressure points to relieve spot areas of tension or muscle pain.

Overall, many people find massage helpful in promoting relaxation and overall well-being at every age.

What Are the Benefits of Chiropractic Care for Menopause?

Chiropractic care is a form of alternative medicine that focuses on the musculoskeletal system, particularly the spine. It aims to improve the health of the musculoskeletal system by correcting spinal "misalignments" via manual manipulations and chiropractic adjustments. The benefits of chiropractic care can include pain relief for the back and neck, improved posture, and improved range of motion of the joints, as well as enhanced flexibility and mobility. Because chiropractic care is specifically focused on the musculoskeletal system, it may play a role in relieving symptoms originating there: muscle pain, back and neck pain, and joint pain and inflammation.

Chiropractic care is not a direct treatment for the hormonal changes of menopause, but it may play a supportive role in relieving some of the physical and functional symptoms that menopausal women may experience.

What Are the Benefits of Herbal Remedies for Menopausal Symptoms?

Herbal remedies have been suggested for everything from hot flashes to hair loss. They generally fall into one of three categories:

» Those that have shown some benefit when it comes to relieving some menopausal symptoms
» Those that have shown no benefit at all
» Those that may even be harmful

Herbs that are called *phytoestrogens* (red clover and soy isoflavones are two examples) have been found in some studies to help with moods and some menopausal symptoms like hot flashes. The ideal doses are unknown, and the studies are generally small, but they don't seem to cause harm at low doses.

Evening primrose oil has been studied in some controlled trials that suggest it may reduce some psychological or mood symptoms, but the evidence for hot flashes is mixed.

Black cohosh, a plant that's native to eastern North America, is a dietary herbal supplement used to reduce vasomotor symptoms like hot flashes and night sweats. Several studies have looked at products that contain black cohosh extracts, alone or in combination with other herbs. Overall, they found that this herb is somewhat beneficial for hot flashes and night sweats but not for symptoms like depression and anxiety. However, black cohosh may cause liver damage in some people. Also, it may relieve hot flashes and night sweats by acting like estrogen, so it has the potential to also act like estrogen on breast tissue and uterine tissue, causing that tissue to be stimulated in the same way that estrogen can stimulate it, possibly causing pre-cancerous or cancerous growth of these cells.

An herb called don quai may act like estrogen in the body and can also increase bleeding risk by thinning the blood.

Kava, an herb often used for anxiety or mood disorders, can cause severe liver damage.

TIP

The rules for making and distributing herbs are much less strict than those for drugs, and they are not regulated or approved by the Food and Drug Administration (FDA). Be sure to talk with your healthcare provider about any herbs you're thinking about taking.

3

Physical Health in Menopause

Chapter **6**
Sexual, Reproductive, and Urinary Health

I n menopause, sexual, reproductive, and urinary health are top concerns. You may wonder how menopause will affect your relationship or sex life, what you can do about vaginal dryness, how your reproductive organs will be affected, or whether you'll still need a pap test after menopause. This chapter answers all these questions and more.

How Does Menopause Affect Relationships and Intimacy?

Usually, in menopause, when hormones are waning, the drive for intimacy may decrease as well. Hormones, like estrogen and testosterone drive desire and arousal, so it may take a little more work and planning to continue to have a robust intimate connection. Long-term relationships may get into a rut; women in menopause may feel that the spark is gone, but there are many ways to make sure the fire doesn't go out. Medications, hormones, therapy, planning, and education are all available to help maintain relationships and intimacy throughout menopause.

How Does Menopause Affect Sexual Health?

Menopause can affect sexual health in many ways. Physically, many changes begin to occur when estrogen production starts to decline. The tissues that are very estrogen-responsive, like vaginal, vulvar, and bladder tissues may undergo menopausal changes due to lack of estrogen. Skin may become thin and dry; vaginal and vulvar tissues will have decreased blood flow and may lose their elasticity and lubrication. When vaginal tissues become dry and thin, sex may become difficult, painful, or impossible. The good news is that creams, suppositories, and even oral medications can work to replace estrogen in these most sensitive tissues and can help restore moisture, elasticity, sensitivity, and congestion, relieving pain and discomfort. Lubricants and warming gels can effectively increase blood flow and congestion, making sexual activity more comfortable and enjoyable.

Sexual health comprises so much more than just vaginal or genital health; it includes moods and mental health, sexual thoughts, interest, libido, and relationship patterns. In menopause there may be changes in body image and self-perception as weight, skin, and hair undergo the changes of menopause. If there is a change in libido, or sexual problems related to hot flashes or night sweats, considering menopausal hormone therapy including testosterone may help.

TIP

Sex therapists or counselors can help with the psychological and emotional aspects of decreased desire and changes in relationship dynamics.

How Does Menopause Affect Libido?

Libido is defined as a person's overall drive or desire for sexual activity. It can have many influences and can naturally vary over time. In the past, scientists thought that libido had to be spontaneous to be "normal," but more recently, for women, the concept of a *responsive libido* has been introduced. Responsive libido is the desire that awakens *after* some stimulus is introduced;

touch, emotional connection, or visual stimulus may stimulate arousal, and desire can follow. As hormone levels diminish in menopause, especially estrogen and testosterone, libido may also decline over time, especially with age or in long-term relationships. Aside from hormones, interest in and desire for sex is influenced by mood and mental health, physical health and body self-image, as well as relationship dynamics, medications and life stressors. It isn't a given or expected that women in menopause should "naturally" have less interest in sex.

Sexual desire in women is a complex issue, incorporating physical and mental health, hormonal health as well as relationship issues. Sometimes, in long-term relationships or with aging, desire that was previously present may diminish or vanish completely. In menopause, with the decrease in hormones and the effect of diminished hormone production on the body (poor sleep, symptomatic hot flashes, vaginal dryness) libido may seem to naturally lessen as time goes on. Evaluating the history of the declining libido and addressing the various components of diminishing desire can lead to a successful return of either spontaneous or responsive desire.

How Can I Increase My Libido If It's Disappearing?

In some women, counseling or therapy may help change the way they view their libido or sexual interest. In others, taking medications that are approved to boost libido (such as flibanserin and bremelanotide) or off-label medications that have been found to boost libido in certain circumstances (such as buspirone and testosterone) may be the solution.

Scientists once thought that low testosterone was the cause of low libido in menopausal women, but studies have found that not to be accurate; testosterone levels start to decline in women in their late 30s and continue to diminish through perimenopause and menopause. Many women who have low testosterone levels have normal libidos. Some studies have even found testosterone levels in women may increase again in their 60s. Although there is not a direct proven correlation between taking testosterone (which is not approved by the Food and Drug Administration [FDA] to treat women's low libido) and increasing libido, some studies have reported that women feel increased interest, desire, and arousal after taking testosterone. There is some evidence about the safety of certain doses and routes of administration. In September 2019, a Global Statement on Testosterone Therapy in Women was published, reviewing the use and dosing of testosterone as an evidence-based guideline for clinicians.

TIP

Most important is finding a physician or practitioner who has been trained in safe and effective ways to evaluate, diagnose, and properly treat symptoms of low libido because many medications and hormones can have side effects that may be unexpected or irreversible.

Some things that may help include:

» Stress management
» Hormone therapy (including testosterone)
» Relationship or sexual therapy
» Cognitive behavioral therapy (CBT)
» Mindfulness
» Medications specifically prescribed for low libido

A plan to relieve vaginal dryness so sex is more comfortable may also help feelings of desire, arousal, and sexual interest.

Can Menopause Cause Vaginal Dryness and Discomfort?

Vaginal (internal) and vulvar (external) tissues are very estrogen sensitive. In menopause (or in any other condition where estrogen levels are low or zero), these tissues can become dry, thin, and inelastic. There can be actual contraction and shrinkage of the tissues, causing discomfort and pain. All of this can make sex difficult or impossible. Plus, lack of estrogen to this area can affect bladder function, causing leakage, irritation, and frequent urinary infections.

Vaginal dryness in menopause is the one menopausal symptom that will require some type of ongoing treatment for the long term to maintain comfort and function. Continuous use of some type of menopausal vaginal treatment is the best way to relieve dryness and discomfort in the genital area, and this should be thought of as a "forever" treatment plan.

What Is Available for Vaginal Dryness in Menopause?

Dryness of the vaginal tissues (and the external skin on the vulva) can be treated with several different categories of products and medications. If the only symptom that the dryness is causing is pain with sexual activity, various lubricants may relieve this symptom. Lubricants are either water-based or silicone-based; each has its own benefits. Water-based lubricants are thinner, are easier to clean up, and can be used with silicone sex toys. Silicone lubes are thicker, but may stain bedsheets, and can't be used with silicone sex toys.

TIP

Lubricants work to relieve dryness and discomfort *only* at the time of a sexual encounter. They aren't long-lasting and they don't permanently change the vaginal tissues in any way.

Vaginal moisturizers can be used as lubricants for sexual activity, but they can also be used for providing longer-lasting vaginal moisture and comfort for up to three days. Don't use products with alcohol, fragrance, perfumes, or dyes added (read the ingredients!) because those can all be irritants to vaginal tissues. Vaginal moisturizers can be purchased online or over the counter and do not contain hormones. Many products contain hyaluronic acid, which is actually an effective moisturizer for vaginal tissues, keeping the vaginal pH at a healthy low level. (Some examples are HYALO-GYN, RepHresh, Replens, Revaree, and Via.)

TIP

The gold standard for women who would like to relieve vaginal dryness, irritation, pain, and burning that accompany menopause (referred to as *genitourinary syndrome of menopause*) is local hormone therapy. Topical estrogen, used in and around the vagina, not only works on vaginal dryness but also changes the elasticity, thickness, and congestion in the genital area for as long as it's used. Estrogen, which can be applied to the genital area comes in a cream, a suppository, a small vaginal pill, and a silicone ring. All are effective in relieving vaginal symptoms, and creams can also be applied to the external skin. They all require a prescription from a healthcare provider, along with instructions for frequency of use. There is also a suppository made of an adrenal hormone called dehydroepiandrosterone (DHEA), which is placed nightly in the vagina; once it melts, it metabolizes into estrogen and testosterone. It's also available by prescription.

In menopause, topical products are usually recommended for vaginal dryness symptoms, but some women use oral medications to relieve vaginal dryness. These also require a prescription and a discussion of medical history and possible side effects.

How Do Hormones Impact Genital Tissues?

In menopause, any tissues that are stimulated by and responsive to, hormones will change when those hormones are gone. The genital tissues (vagina, vulvar skin, and even the bladder) are affected in a positive way by the presence of estrogen — it keeps those tissues healthy and moist and maintains congestion and blood flow. In menopause, when there is no more estrogen present, the tissues become dry and lose some of their elasticity. The bladder can become more irritable, and the vaginal and vulvar tissues can become thin and uncomfortable.

Replacing the local loss of estrogen with creams, gels, suppositories, or tablets can help restore moisture and the normal texture and elasticity to these tissues. These prescription medications actually change dry tissue over time and help with discomfort and irritation in the genital area.

Vaginal estrogen creams are usually recommended to be applied inside the vagina (and sometimes externally) two to three times a week at bedtime. Some women find the creams a bit messy and prefer to use other types of estrogen. A suppository or vaginal estrogen pill can also be prescribed to be used two to three times per week at bedtime; they melt at body temperature, working overnight so by the morning there isn't much mess. The vaginal ring stays in the vagina for 90 days at a time, emitting a continuous small amount of estrogen for three months, after which it's removed and replaced immediately by another ring. Women who would rather not think about daily, weekly, or twice-weekly vaginal treatments may be good candidates for the ring.

How Does Menopause Affect Reproductive Organs?

Reproductive organs are the parts of the body involved in sexual reproduction. The biggest change during menopause is that the ovaries, which have been responsible for producing hormones like estrogen, progesterone, and testosterone for many years, stop functioning. Ovulation also stops completely in menopause. Usually, over time, the ovaries may become smaller after they're no longer functioning.

Other reproductive organs include the uterus and cervix, which don't change much in menopause, other than no longer functioning as the location where menstrual blood would collect monthly in preparation for a monthly period. In menopause, no blood will collect and there should be no bleeding.

The vagina does change in menopause because the vaginal tissues are responsive to estrogen and need estrogen to stay healthy. In menopause, when estrogen is no longer being produced, vaginal tissues can become thin and dry. Using local estrogen or other moisturizers in the vaginal area can help increase blood flow and maintain moisture and elasticity.

How Does Menopause Affect Reproductive Cycles?

The very definition of *menopause* is the cessation of ovarian function. When the ovaries stop working, they stop producing hormones and stop ovulating. When there is no hormone production and no ovulation, there will be no further menstrual cycles and should be no further bleeding.

Sometimes the years preceding menopause can be a time of very irregular hormone production, and there may be lots of hormone swings and irregular bleeding. This is typical of perimenopause. However, after menopause is diagnosed (12 consecutive months without a period) there should be no further bleeding and no cycling.

How Does Menopause Impact Reproductive Hormones?

In menopause, the levels of reproductive hormones (estrogen, progesterone, and testosterone) should be low or close to zero. The ovaries, where most estrogen (also called estradiol) is made and where most progesterone is produced are not functioning in menopause, so very little of these hormones will be found in the body. These hormones can be made in small amounts in other organs in the body, though. The adrenal glands, located on top of the kidneys, produce dehydroepiandrosterone (DHEA), which is a hormone that can be converted into estrogen in various tissues. After menopause, *adipose* (fatty) tissue converts androgens (like testosterone) into estrogen, and very small amounts of estrogen can be produced in the liver and brain. The adrenal glands and the brain can also produce very small amounts of progesterone.

Testosterone is produced about 50 percent in the ovaries and 50 percent in the adrenal glands, so after menopause, there still will be some circulating testosterone in the body.

The small amount of estrogen produced or present in menopause is a different type than the type produced by the ovaries in younger years, and not enough to keep women from having hot flashes and night sweats.

How Does Menopause Impact Urinary Health?

Lack of estrogen in menopause negatively impacts vaginal tissue and bladder tissue. There are many estrogen receptors in these areas, and the vaginal walls become dry and thin without estrogen. This can lead to vaginal discomfort, as well as bladder problems: urine leakage, urinary urgency, and urinary tract infections. The good news is that using topical estrogen vaginally (which comes in many forms) can bring back moisture, congestion, and health to the genitourinary tissues and correct or eliminate these problems.

Do I Still Need a Pap Smear in Menopause?

A pap test (or "smear" as it used to be called) is a screening test for cervical cancer. There are guidelines from medical societies on when and if certain women, or certain populations of women, need this screening test and if so, how often.

Almost all abnormal pap tests that show precancer (also called dysplasia) or cervical cancers are caused by a particular virus, called the human papilloma virus (HPV). HPV is the most common of all the sexually transmitted viruses; about 70 percent of all people who have been sexually active have at some point contracted this virus and may be carriers. Most women who contract HPV will never be diagnosed with cancer or precancer, but some will, and screening intervals are based on risk.

In menopause, up to age 65, if a woman is low risk (hasn't had abnormal pap smears in the past, is not suffering from immune suppression, and has no symptoms), pap tests are usually repeated about every three to five years, possibly changing the interval if health conditions change or if new sexual partners are introduced. After age 65, pap tests are usually only done if there is a risk that something abnormal may be found (if an exam is abnormal, if there is bleeding, or if there is a past history of precancer or cancer of the cervix or genital area). If there are no new sexual partners, it is unlikely that an HPV-related abnormality will be newly found in a previously negative woman in menopause.

TIP

The decision on whether to do a pap test should be an individual assessment based on risk and guidelines; a healthcare provider should always explain why you do or do not need to repeat another pap test as you age.

Chapter **7**

Metabolism and the Endocrine System

M enopause brings about significant shifts in metabolism and the endocrine system. The results can include a slower metabolism (and weight gain, especially around the midsection), increased insulin resistance (and greater risk of diabetes), and redistribution of fat. This chapter walks you through the metabolic and endocrine changes that are common during menopause so you know what to expect and how to handle them.

How Does Menopause Affect Metabolic Health?

Menopause brings with it a shift in metabolic health that is driven mostly by the drop in estrogen. Body fat tends to redistribute from the hips and thighs to the abdomen. This "middle fat" brings increased health risks with it. If you don't make a concerted effort to maintain muscle mass with a concentration on protein in the diet and regular resistance training, you'll lose lean muscle mass and gain more fatty tissue. This may be accompanied by a higher low-density lipoprotein (LDL) cholesterol level and an increased risk for cardiovascular disease.

The *basal metabolic rate* (the rate at which the body burns calories just from doing normal everyday activities) often declines with age and with decreased estrogen and progesterone, leading to slower calorie burning. Fat distribution often shifts at this time, causing weight gain specifically in the abdomen rather than in the hips and thighs.

Can Menopause Cause Changes in Blood Sugar Levels?

Estrogen increases the sensitivity to insulin in the muscles and liver. (Insulin, made by the pancreas, helps the body to metabolize sugar and utilize it in the body's cells.) Estrogen helps the cells take in glucose more efficiently, which can help keep blood sugar levels stable. In menopause, when estrogen levels decline, cells may become more resistant to insulin. Fasting glucose levels generally rise after menopause, and the risk of diabetes increases. Also, after menopause, fat tends to collect in the abdominal area; this type of fat is more resistant to insulin.

Can Menopause Increase Risk for Diabetes?

Diabetes is a medical condition in which the pancreas, which produces insulin to help the body use sugar from food and send it into the body's cells to be used for energy, doesn't work efficiently or at all. When the pancreas doesn't effectively make insulin, the sugar level in the bloodstream will be high, which can lead to many medical complications.

Prediabetes is the condition that often occurs before the pancreas has lost much of its function; sugar levels are considered borderline high in this condition.

The risk for prediabetes and diabetes increases in menopause as the effects of declining estrogen are felt at the level of the pancreas. Estrogen assists cells in effectively absorbing glucose. Without estrogen, insulin is less able to act efficiently, so menopausal women often have higher blood sugar levels.

Women who have had many years of weight fluctuations, losing and gaining weight over a period of years, are more at risk for diabetes and prediabetes because weight fluctuations can have a negative effect on the pancreas's ability to efficiently move sugar from the diet into the body's cells.

Can Menopause Cause Changes in Appetite?

Not specific to menopause, but in any time of increased stress or poor sleep, appetite is affected in several ways. You may experience an increase in cravings for unhealthy foods, especially those high in fat and high in sugar (so-called "comfort foods"). There is a hormone produced in the stomach that increases hunger, and this hormone increases if stress or poor sleep occur in menopause.

Experiences vary widely on whether menopause or any hormonal shift actually changes appetite. The decline in estrogen and progesterone is thought to have an influence on hunger cues — it can change appetite and eating habits. A hormone called leptin sends a signal to the brain telling it that you feel full. Drops in estrogen may blunt the effect of leptin, causing increased appetite. There are some other ways that menopause may affect the appetite: poor sleep, stress, and mood changes in menopause can often lead to *comfort eating* (seeking comfort through eating certain foods that are sweet or fatty).

How Does Menopause Affect the Endocrine System?

The endocrine system is composed of the organs of the body that participate in hormonal secretion. This includes the pituitary gland in the brain, the thyroid gland, the adrenal glands (two small glands located on top of the kidneys), the pancreas, and also the adipose (fatty) tissue. The body's hormonal networks are interconnected, so when the ovaries stop functioning (which defines menopause), many changes take place in many other organs.

When estrogen drops, thyroid hormone levels may rise, which can result in fluctuating metabolism and energy, as well as sleep disruption. Chronic stress during menopause can cause the adrenal glands to produce increased amounts of cortisol, which can result in sleep disruption and the accumulation of belly fat. Estrogen normally improves insulin sensitivity, so without it, cells become more insulin resistant, causing blood glucose levels to rise more easily and increasing the risk for type 2 diabetes. Because adrenal hormones like cortisol also rise in times of chronic stress, the recommended solution is to figure out what's causing the stress and try to reduce it. There are no supplements proven to change the way in which the adrenal glands function.

How Does Menopause Affect Thyroid Health?

Menopause and thyroid health can affect each other. Menopause is not thought to directly affect thyroid disease, but many of the hormonal changes of menopause may cause symptoms that are similar to thyroid symptoms. Estrogen can affect the levels of proteins that carry thyroid hormones in the blood. Thyroid disease becomes more common with age, and thyroid medication doses may need to be adjusted based on the use of menopausal hormone therapy.

How Does Menopause Impact Adrenal Health?

Hormones are produced in the body in reproductive years mostly by the ovaries and, to a lesser extent, by the adrenal glands. In menopause, when the ovaries are making little to no estrogen, progesterone, and testosterone, the adrenal glands proportionately produce more hormones. The adrenals produce dehydroepiandrosterone (DHEA) and other precursor hormones, which can be converted to estrogen and testosterone in the body in small amounts. The adrenal glands also produce cortisol, which is a hormone needed in times of stress.

Menopause does not directly shut down or damage the adrenal glands, but after ovarian production of hormones declines, the adrenal glands become the primary source of several hormones (DHEA and testosterone). With this drop in ovarian hormones, the adrenal glands take on relatively greater endocrine responsibility at the same time sleep disruption and hot flashes are occurring. These menopausal stressors may cause an alteration in adrenal regulation, leaving women feeling exhausted yet overstimulated.

How Does Menopause Cause Changes in the Cholesterol Profile?

A basic cholesterol blood panel consists of total cholesterol, high-density lipoprotein (HDL) cholesterol, LDL, and triglycerides. Having an elevated LDL cholesterol level is most closely associated with an increased risk for cardio-vascular disease and stroke. Total cholesterol, triglycerides, and LDL cholesterol often rise in menopause because estrogen has a beneficial effect on the way the liver produces and metabolizes cholesterol; this benefit may be lost with the decline in estrogen.

Women who previously had normal or low cholesterol levels may find that in menopause they need medication to keep their cholesterol in normal ranges, even if they have a healthy diet and exercise. Keeping cholesterol, especially LDL, in normal ranges is very important in menopause when other factors that can increase cardiovascular risk (high blood pressure, weight gain, and diabetes or prediabetes) may be at play.

What Affect Does Menopause Have on Bone-Regulating Hormones?

Estrogen helps regulate the balance between bone builders and bone destroyers in the body. After menopause, bone breakdown increases, placing menopausal women at increased risk for osteoporosis and fractures. This is part of the endocrine impact of menopause. Estrogen governs calcium use in the body, as well as the efficiency with which vitamin D aids in maintaining calcium deposition in the bones. Without estrogen, there is accelerated bone breakdown, and women lose up to 10 percent of their bone mass in the first five years after their final menstrual period.

Chapter **8**
Cardiovascular Health

Among estrogen's many benefits, its support of cardiovascular health is one of the most important. The risk of cardiovascular disease increases by roughly 50 percent in the first five years of menopause. This chapter explains how menopause affects cardiovascular health, what you can do to maintain cardiovascular health in menopause, and how menopause can affect cholesterol and blood pressure.

How Does Menopause Affect Cardiovascular Health?

Estrogen has a protective effect on the heart, lowering inflammation and keeping blood vessels healthy. When estrogen levels fall dramatically, as they do during menopause, the estrogenic protections diminish, increasing the risk for high blood pressure and damage to blood vessel walls, causing clogs and clots, and increasing the risk for heart attacks and strokes. Lower estrogen levels also often lead to a rise in low-density lipoprotein (LDL), which accelerates plaque buildup in the arteries, causing blockages.

How Can I Maintain Heart Health during Menopause?

Maintaining a healthy heart should begin way before menopause — but it's never too late to adopt the healthy habits that help maintain heart health:

» **Pay attention to what you eat.** A healthy diet is important to heart health. Limit processed foods and focus on high-quality, plant-based or lean meat proteins and lots of vegetables.

» **Get enough exercise.** Aim for at least 150 minutes of moderate-intensity activity per week. Include resistance training (with weights, weight machines, or body weight), too.

If you're concerned about "bulking up" like a weightlifter, don't be — It's possible to do enough resistance exercise to maintain lean muscles without the "bulk" of a weightlifter.

» **Quit smoking.** If you smoke, quit. Period.

» **Reduce or eliminate alcohol.** Adopting a low- to no-alcohol habit helps maintain good cardiovascular blood flow and function.

» **Know your cholesterol level, blood pressure, and weight.** Keeping all of these in normal ranges can help minimize stress on the heart.

» **Get enough sleep.** Regularly getting seven to nine hours of good-quality sleep can help overall health and heart health by helping control inflammation.

There is some evidence that women who have hot flashes and night sweats will be healthier if their symptoms are controlled. Hot flashes are increasingly recognized as a marker for cardiovascular disease in midlife women. Hot flashes are associated with more plaque buildup in arteries. Controlling these symptoms in menopause can be important for future heart protection and health. Talk to your healthcare provider about relieving these symptoms if you're transitioning to menopause. "Toughing it out" is not recommended.

How Does Menopause Impact Cholesterol Levels?

Estrogen has cardioprotective effects: It increases high-density lipoprotein (HDL; the "good" cholesterol), decreases LDL ("the bad" cholesterol), and improves the health of blood vessels (vascular function). When estrogen levels drop at menopause, the protective effects of estrogen are lost. Usually (and especially in the first few years into menopause), cholesterol levels and triglycerides will rise. These changes increase vascular disease and increase the risk for heart attacks and strokes.

Can Menopause Cause Changes in Blood Pressure?

Estrogen plays a key role in keeping blood vessels flexible, elastic, responsive, and protected from inflammation. When estrogen declines, blood vessels become stiffer and less able to expand. When vessels become less elastic, blood pressure will often begin to rise. The inner lining of the blood vessels, called the *endothelium*, is very sensitive to estrogen; without estrogen, the endothelium is more likely to become inflamed and allow for the buildup of plaque. The resting heart rate can rise as the heart has to pump harder to pump blood through these vessels; this can lead to a sense of "jitteriness" or palpitations that many menopausal women report. When blood vessels become less elastic and it's harder for the heart to pump blood through them, blood pressure may rise, and cardiovascular risk accelerates.

Chapter **9**
Systemic Health

Menopause has effects throughout the body, not just the reproductive system or cardiovascular system. Scientists are just starting to understand the links between estrogen, progesterone, and the gastrointestinal microbiome; this chapter covers what we know so far. It also fills you in on liver and kidney health, how menopause affects the immune system and respiratory system, and more.

Can Menopause Increase the Risk of Certain Cancers?

Cancer usually develops from a combination of lifestyle, genetic, environmental, infectious, and hormonal factors. The risk of many cancers increases with age, so menopause can be a time when age plus the many cumulative contributors may come together.

Smoking and excess alcohol intake are risk factors for cancers like liver, throat, breast, lung, and colon cancer. A diet high in processed, fatty, or smoked foods increases the risk of colon and other gastrointestinal cancers. A sedentary lifestyle and excess body fat increase the risk of breast, colon, and endometrial (uterine) cancers. A strong family history of breast, ovarian, pancreatic, uterine, or colon cancer may prompt a genetic test to look for mutations in DNA. Having a genetic mutation greatly increases the chance that a person will be diagnosed with one of these cancers.

Going into menopause much later than average (which is age 51) slightly increases the lifetime estrogen exposure, which may increase your risk for a hormone-sensitive cancer, such as endometrial or breast cancer.

Some cancers, like cervical cancer, are caused by infections. The human papilloma virus (HPV) is implicated in cervical, vulvar, anal, esophageal, and throat cancers. As women age, their immune systems are less capable of fighting off HPV and other viruses, so women in menopause with a history of having HPV may need to continue to be screened for cervical cancer with pap smears and pelvic exams.

How Does Menopause Affect Gastrointestinal Health?

Gastroesophageal reflux disease (GERD) is more common in menopause because estrogen helps in maintaining the tone of the *esophageal sphincter* (the muscle at the lower end of the esophagus). When muscle tone decreases, you may experience more of a reflux of stomach contents, causing *acidic* (burning) symptoms.

Menopausal women who take oral forms of estrogen have a higher incidence of gallstones and gallbladder problems.

Also, estrogen and progesterone may help maintain intestinal motility so a decline in these hormones can increase the risk of constipation.

What Are Some Common Gastrointestinal Symptoms Associated with Menopause?

The stomach, intestines, and liver have receptors for estrogen and progesterone. A decline in these hormones in menopause causes many potential changes throughout the gastrointestinal tract. The mouth can get dry, changing the speed with which food is digested, and *motility* (the rate at which food passes through the digestive system) slows down. The type of bacteria present in the stomach and intestines can change, reducing the number and type of beneficial bacterial species.

Common gastrointestinal symptoms in menopause include:

>> Bloating

>> Constipation

>> Acid reflux

>> Worsening of inflammatory bowel conditions

>> Changes in frequency of bowel movements

Although some of these symptoms may be related specifically to the decrease in hormones, other menopausal symptoms like poor sleep and increased stress also can have an influence on the G.I. tract and intestinal activity.

TIP

To maintain good gastrointestinal health in menopause, the focus should be on increased hydration and adequate fiber intake (vegetables, beans, seeds, oats, and fruit) at every meal. Some people feel intake of fermented foods (like yogurt, kefir, sauerkraut, miso, and kimchi) also helps with healthy gastrointestinal function because they may improve the gut microbiome.

How Does Menopause Affect Respiratory Health?

Menopause doesn't have many widely recognized effects on lung function. However, in women with asthma or other respiratory or airway diseases, a lack of estrogen can result in a worsening of respiratory function. Declines in lung function may be just a part of normal aging, so the incidence of conditions like obstructive sleep apnea or asthma may increase after menopause.

The way in which menopause affects the respiratory system is not often studied or reported on. Estrogen and progesterone affect elasticity in other tissues, so the decline in these hormones can also affect the elasticity of lung tissue. Having adequate estrogen and progesterone also helps minimize inflammation in the body, and if lung tissue becomes inflamed, lung capacity and efficiency can be slightly compromised. Some women may feel symptoms of shortness of breath in menopause, which may not be directly related to diminishing hormones but may be connected to other menopausal symptoms, like anxiety or hot flashes.

Sometimes, there is an onset of new lung disease in menopause, such as asthma or chronic obstructive pulmonary disease (COPD), but scientists don't know if these new disorders are related to menopause itself or due to a combination of health changes that occur at this time (weight gain, occupational exposures, smoking history, and emergence of autoimmune diseases).

How Does Menopause Impact Liver Health?

Menopausal women have a much higher incidence of liver disease than younger women. Estrogen influences the amount of fat that accumulates in the liver, and when there is a lack of estrogen, there may be more fat in the liver, leading to something called fatty liver disease.

How Does Menopause Affect Kidney Health?

The kidneys depend on many small blood vessels functioning correctly to be able to filter waste and fluid from the blood and produce urine. Estrogen has a protective effect on blood vessels, and when estrogen levels decline, blood vessels are more likely to be inflamed. Inflamed blood vessels are less efficient, and this, combined with other conditions that are more likely to appear as we age (high blood pressure, diabetes) can cause a decrease in the efficient functioning of the kidneys.

Estrogen's protective effect on the kidneys is not conclusive, but some data suggests that estrogen therapy, if started prior to the decrease in kidney function, may decrease inflammation and provide benefit.

How Does Menopause Affect Oral Health?

Menopause can affect oral health by causing dry mouth. Saliva washes away food particles and bacteria and neutralizes acid from food.

Producing less saliva can lead to gum disease, cavities, and pain.

Hormones, especially estrogen, are thought to have a protective effect on nerve function. Some menopausal women experience burning and pain in the mouth, also called burning mouth syndrome.

Can Menopause Cause Changes in Body Odor?

When a lack of estrogen causes hot flashes, body temperature rises and can cause more daytime and nighttime sweating. This increased sweating can occur especially in the glands under the arms and in the groin. There are proteins in this area that can be broken down by bacteria, which can cause odor to be released with the sweat. Of course, odor with perspiration can occur at any age, but in menopause, with a decrease in estrogen, there can be higher levels of *androgens* (male hormones) by comparison, which can change the way sweat smells.

Many women notice changes in their body odor in menopause. The changes may be linked to alterations in the *skin microbiome* (the types of bacteria that naturally live on the skin), temperature regulation, hormones, and the composition of the sweat. As estrogen levels fall, sweat glands become more active as the temperature regulation area of the brain changes. The composition of sweat changes, with increased sodium, more proteins, more ammonia, and more odor-producing bacteria.

The general effect of these changes is to produce a stronger, muskier-scented sweat, containing more odor-producing bacteria. This has less to do with hygiene and more to do with declining or absent levels of estrogen. Limiting spicy foods, red meat, and ultra-processed foods and maintaining adequate hydration can help change the components of sweat. Using wipes with gentle lactic acid cleansers in the groin and underarm areas may help maintain the skin's natural acidity and help suppress bacteria-produced odor.

How Does Menopause Affect the Immune System?

Estrogen and progesterone have an impact on inflammation in the body and how the body responds to new infections. The loss of these hormones causes a decrease in the number and function of antibodies produced by the body (cells that fight off inflammation and infection) resulting in more chronic inflammation and slower immune responses. Menopausal women also may have a less-than-robust reaction to new vaccines, possibly making them less effective.

Autoimmune diseases like lupus, Sjögren's syndrome, and rheumatoid arthritis may become more noticeable or flare in menopause, but this isn't necessarily related directly to menopause.

However, when estrogen levels fall, baseline inflammation rises, and inflammatory markers can cause symptoms to flare.

What Are the Best Ways to Manage Menopause-Related Fatigue?

Fatigue, a feeling of ongoing exhaustion, is one of the most common and frustrating complaints at any time of life, but in some women, it seems to worsen and become more pronounced in perimenopause and menopause. Fatigue can be from many contributing factors (physical, mental, and emotional), and it's often a combination. It's essential to determine the possible causes for menopause-related fatigue, because treating this symptom relies on finding and treating the root cause.

TIP

Treatable medical conditions should be ruled out first, by evaluating for thyroid disease, anemia, vitamin or iron deficiencies, auto-immune conditions, and diabetes, to name a few. A healthcare practitioner should be able to decide which of these or other tests can be done to diagnose a medical condition that can be causing feelings of fatigue.

After medical conditions are treated or ruled out, other sources of fatigue should be investigated. Poor sleep quality, including limited deep or restorative sleep, can cause daytime fatigue.

A sleep study or just a history of sleep hygiene and habits can be undertaken to see if correcting behaviors or using a continuous positive airway pressure (CPAP) machine may be needed to get better length and quality of sleep.

Stress, anxiety, depression, or other mental health issues if undiagnosed or unrecognized can cause feelings of fatigue. Chronic stress maintains the body in a constant feeling of high alert, which can result in feelings of fatigue. Stress management, counseling, cognitive behavioral therapy (CBT), and various medications can treat mental health issues and go a long way toward reducing feelings of fatigue and exhaustion.

If it seems the feelings of fatigue began or suddenly worsened with the onset of menopause, and other causes have been eliminated, menopausal hormone therapy, though not a direct treatment for fatigue, may help to improve sleep, reduce anxiety, and add to an overall feeling of well-being in some people.

TIP

If fatigue is sudden, severe, or worsening or if you have unexplained weight loss or heart palpitations along with the fatigue, see your doctor right away. These symptoms may signal a more severe medical condition.

How Does Menopause Affect Musculoskeletal Health?

Possible effects of menopause on the musculoskeletal system include:

- » Bone loss and increased risk for osteoporosis and fracture
- » Joint stiffness, swelling, and aches
- » Loss of muscle mass and strength
- » Changes in connective tissues

Estrogen is a protector of muscle, bone, and joint function, and when that protection is lost, joints tend to become stiffer and possibly more inflamed, muscle tends to get weaker, and bones can get thin.

Keeping active in perimenopause and in menopause can be helpful by maintaining muscle strength and bone density. Estrogen is indicated for prevention of osteoporosis if it's started early in menopause; it can also help to reduce bone fractures.

TIP

Balance and weight-bearing exercises and activity, if done regularly, can have an impact on musculoskeletal health way into the menopause years.

How Can I Best Treat Balance Problems in Menopause?

Some menopausal women begin to experience problems with balance. This is usually from a combination of factors:

- » Changes in muscle mass
- » Sleep disruptions

» Weight gain

» Vision and/or hearing changes

» Loss of protection that estrogen provided to the vestibular system (which helps with balance)

A combination approach to treating balance problems is probably best. Stretching, doing lower-body and core strengthening exercises, engaging in regular weight-bearing physical activity, addressing any changes in vision and/or hearing, and taking anti-inflammatory medications can all contribute to treating balance issues.

TIP

Single-leg timed standing, heel-and-toe walking, and tai chi have all been shown to help for balance and fall prevention.

Chapter **10**
Bones, Muscles, and Joints

Women typically lose about 10 percent of their bone density in the first five years of menopause. This chapter covers everything to do with bones, muscles, and joints and what you can do to protect them.

How Much Does Menopause Affect Bone Health?

Due to the decline in estrogen levels in menopause, bone loss accelerates. Estrogen has a slowing effect on the rate of *bone resorption* (the rate at which bone is broken down). The rate of bone loss is fastest in the first few years in menopause. Without estrogen, new bone can't be made. *Osteopenia* (slight bone loss) and *osteoporosis* (more major bone loss) become more common after menopause, and bones are at higher risk for fracture.

Can Menopause Cause Joint Pain and Stiffness?

Women in menopause often have more joint pain and stiffness, but the reasons are not fully understood. Scientists think that estrogen may play a protective role in the health of joints and connective tissue, but inactivity, aging, and medical conditions can all play a role. There are estrogen receptors in joints, so it's possible that estrogen directly affects these tissues. Without estrogen, there may be more inflammation, leading to more joint swelling and discomfort. Other factors, like reduced physical activity, poor sleep, and weight gain, can also influence pain, swelling, and inflammation of the joints, so moving is key!

Can Menopause Cause Changes in Muscle Mass and Strength?

Muscle mass, and subsequently, a loss of strength, happens for many different reasons in menopause. Aging, lifestyle changes, and hormonal shifts can all combine to cause the loss of lean muscle. A decrease in activity, especially resistance exercises (using weights, weight machines, or body weight), accelerates muscle loss. Decreased estrogen weakens muscle maintenance and the ability of muscles to repair themselves.

Estrogen plays a large role in muscle mass, strength, and repair. When estrogen levels decline, women can lose up to 8 percent of muscle mass each decade of life after age 40. When there is a loss in lean muscle mass, there is also usually a gain in weight, especially in the adipose (fatty) tissue that accumulates in the abdomen.

TIP

These muscle changes can be prevented by doing resistance training three to four times per week and taking in an adequate amount of healthy protein. Adequate protein intake for most menopausal women is considered to be approximately 1 to 1.2 grams of protein per kilogram of body weight per day. (You can find your approximate weight in kilograms by dividing your weight in pounds by 2.205 — or just use your favorite search engine to search the web for "pounds to kilograms.")

Aging in general causes a loss of muscle mass, and when estrogen drops, the breakdown of muscle protein increases. It's harder to build new muscle in menopause, and women lose much more muscle mass in the years immediately after the menopausal transition. If physical activity decreases (exercise, especially resistance exercises), women will lose muscle mass and muscle tone. Muscle fibers shrink, and the power of the muscle is reduced, leading to difficulty in climbing, lifting, and reacting quickly to prevent a fall.

Can I Take Supplements to Help Build New Muscle?

Creatine is a naturally occurring compound the body makes from amino acids. It's stored in muscle cells to be used as an energy source for bursts of activity. Some studies have shown that taking a creatine supplement may help women increase muscle strength and lean mass, but only when it's combined with vigorous resistance training. In studies of menopausal women, creatine appeared to be safe, with few adverse side effects. The usual dose is 3 to 5 grams per day.

Protein supplementation has been shown to improve lean mass and muscle strength in older women, but, like creatine, only if it's combined with vigorous resistance training. Studies have shown that protein supplementation alone has little to no benefit for midlife and older women. For very active women, or those who struggle to get enough protein through their diet (which is what most experts recommend as the source of protein), a protein supplement or shake can fill the gap.

What Kind of Supplements Can Help Menopausal Bones?

Supplements are not a substitute for resistance training, weight-bearing exercise, and healthy nutrition, but several supplements are commonly thought to help support menopausal bone health.

Calcium is the main mineral in bone, you can get it from a diet that includes dairy; green, leafy vegetables; and calcium-fortified foods. The body absorbs the calcium in dairy products well. Some seafood (sardines, salmon, and mackerel) has calcium.

You may need to take a calcium supplement if you're not getting enough calcium through your diet (approximately 1,000 milligrams per day for women over 55).

Vitamin D is important because it aids in the absorption of calcium. It's difficult to get enough vitamin D from foods, because only fatty fish, egg yolks, cod liver oil, and certain fortified foods have vitamin D. The dose you take should be individualized based on your level of risk and the amount of sun exposure you get, because ultraviolet (UV) light triggers vitamin D production in the body.

TIP

If you're considering supplementing with vitamin D, talk to your doctor about whether a supplement is right for you and, if so, how much.

Chapter **11**

Skin, Hair, and Nails

Changes to other systems in the body are sometimes subtle, but most women going through menopause will be able to point to changes in their skin, hair, and nails. This chapter fills you in on exactly how menopause impacts all three and how you can manage related symptoms.

How Does Menopause Impact Skin?

Menopausal women may experience dryness or itching of the skin and scalp, slower wound healing, and decreased oil and sweat. The skin may begin to show dark spots or redness, as well as visible blood vessels and bruising. This happens due to the decrease in estrogen and progesterone, which are two hormones that influence collagen production, elasticity of the skin, and blood flow.

Estrogen helps maintain hydration of the skin, as well as collagen and elastin, which are proteins that maintain the structure and elasticity of the skin and connective tissues. The loss of these proteins leads to thinner, more fragile skin and wrinkles. The skin can also become very sensitive in menopause due to the reduction in circulation and hydration.

Moisturizers like hyaluronic acid and ceramides, as well as retinoids, may help with thin menopausal skin. Wearing sunscreen on any sun-exposed skin is a *must* at any age.

How Does Menopause Affect Hair?

Estrogen also helps to keep hair in a growth phase, also known as the *anagen phase*. In menopause, lower estrogen and relatively higher androgen (male hormone) activity shorten the anagen phase. The shedding phase, known as the *telogen phase*, is longer and the growth phase is shorter. Fewer hairs remain in the active growth phase, so there is more noticeable shedding and slower replacement. The decline of estrogen can lead to thinning of the hair, as well as scalp symptoms like dryness and itching. Many menopausal women notice hair loss on the sides and top of the scalp. Genetics, stress, and medical conditions like thyroid disorders, as well as nutritional deficiencies, can amplify the thinning.

TIP

Good nutrition, menopausal hormone therapy, and prescription medications may all play a role in maintaining the health of the scalp and hair follicles.

How Can I Best Take Care of Menopausal Skin?

TIP

For a menopausal skin routine, consider the following:

» **Morning**

- **Cleanser:** The cleanser should be gentle. No harsh soaps and nothing that contains alcohol. Look for a cleanser with words like *hydrating* and *gentle* on the label. Ingredients like ceramides and hyaluronic acid are good.

- **Hydrating serum:** Look for one containing hyaluronic acid, niacinamide, and/or vitamin C in some combination.

- **Moisturizer:** Look for a nongreasy barrier lotion.

- **Sunscreen:** Aim for a sunscreen with at least SPF 30. (*SPF* stands for *sun protection factor.*)

» Evening

- **Cleanser:** The cleanser can be the same as the one you use in the morning.
- **Treatment serum:** Look for a retinoid serum — they're available over the counter and by prescription. Retinoids are a derivative of vitamin A. They can boost cell turnover and increase collagen production.
- **Moisturizer:** Look for a moisturizer that's thicker than the one you use in the morning. It should provide an overnight barrier.

You can add a hydrating mask once a week to boost moisture. Look for one made with hyaluronic acid or aloe.

TIP

Drinking enough water and getting enough restorative sleep also contribute to an effective menopausal skin care routine.

How Can Menopause Cause Changes in Skin Pigmentation?

In menopause the skin may undergo many changes, related to aging, lifestyle, and a decline in estrogen. Estrogen interacts with the *melanocytes* (pigment-producing cells in the skin). When there is adequate estrogen, skin tone will appear more even, but as estrogen declines, the activity of melanocytes becomes less stable. Some areas of skin, especially sun-exposed skin, will overproduce melanin, which leads to *hyperpigmentation* (dark spots). Other areas will produce too little melanin, leading to *hypopigmentation* (white spots). Skin tone becomes uneven, especially on the face, neck, and hands.

The skin also becomes thinner and has less collagen, making dark spots appear more prominent. Avoid sun exposure and always have barrier protection on sun-exposed skin. Also be sure to wear broad-spectrum sunscreen even on cloudy days and reapply when sweating or swimming.

TIP

Procedures like peels and laser therapy, as well as topical treatments like vitamin C and retinoids, may help fade dark spots and suppress melanin production to help produce a brighter and more even complexion over time.

What Are the Best Ways to Manage Menopausal Hair Loss?

Hundreds of supplements are advertised to restore hair after menopausal hair loss. Many of the studies in support of these supplements have been conducted by the same companies that sell them, so it may be impossible to gauge the veracity of their claims.

Hair loss in menopause is caused by a combination of factors: aging, genetics, lifestyle, nutrition, scalp health, and hydration status.

Eating a healthy and varied diet and staying well hydrated are the most basic components needed for keeping hair healthy. Your healthcare provider may want to check for a thyroid disorder or for nutritional deficiencies (like vitamin D and iron). Some women have found that menopausal hormone therapy improves hair loss, but taking hormones to treat hair loss, without any other indication, is not currently recommended.

Topical minoxidil applied to the scalp has been shown to be helpful in slowing or limiting hair loss; it also helps to grow new hair. An oral preparation of minoxidil is available. Oral finasteride has also showed some benefit for women (not all of whom were in menopause) in stopping hair loss and helping with new growth. These are both prescription medications that require a medical evaluation. Often, effective treatments for hair thinning and loss need to be continued long term; discontinuing their use may result in a resumption of the loss.

Can Menopause Cause Changes in Nail Health?

Estrogen is associated with efficient blood flow, so in menopause, where the blood flow to extremities (like hands and feet) may slow down, nails may grow more slowly and may be slower to repair if broken or damaged. Other factors also contribute to nail health, like nutrition and hydration.

Estrogen plays a role in hydration and collagen production, which are important in nail health. Without estrogen, nails may grow more slowly and become thinner and more brittle, splitting and breaking more easily. Other factors may make nails more fragile, including nutritional deficiencies, environmental exposures like harsh chemicals, and dehydration.

The drop of estrogen in menopause can cause thinning and cracking of the nails. When estrogen levels decline, there is also a decrease in *keratin* (which provides strength and flexibility to the nails) and lipid content in nails. Some nails get lines or ridges in them when they become thinner.

TIP

In menopause, nails should be moisturized daily with oils or moisturizers made specifically for nails and cuticles. You can also protect your nails by wearing gloves when you're working with chemicals or when you're cleaning or gardening. Make sure your diet contains enough protein, zinc, iron, and vitamin D to help nails grow and stay healthy.

What Lifestyle Strategies Can Help Menopausal Skin, Hair, and Nails?

Daily habits are most important. Staying out of direct sunlight as much as possible, and wearing adequate sunscreen for protection can help slow the sun's effects on aging skin. Avoiding tight or pulling hairstyles and harsh chemicals on the hair and scalp may help slow hair loss. Allowing nails to "breathe" without polish on them may help reduce damage and nail breakage.

Nutrition, with adequate protein and vitamin D intake, may help limit the changes seen in menopause. Hydration, mostly with water, will help skin maintain its moisture.

Menopausal hormone therapy is not specifically recommended to remedy skin or hair problems in menopause, but sometimes women using systemic hormones find that there are benefits to skin texture and elasticity or a decrease in hair loss. There are face and skin creams reported to contain estrogen, but these have not been studied in large trials so it's unknown whether they're helpful or safe on a large scale.

Why Might Menopausal Women Find an Increase in Facial or Body Hair but Thinner Scalp Hair?

There are two categories of hormones normally produced in the body: estrogens (considered "female" hormones because they promote what would be considered female characteristics) and androgens ("male" hormones that stimulate more male-type features). Prior to menopause, estrogen is the dominant hormone type that women produce, mostly in the ovaries. When estrogen levels drop in menopause, androgen-sensitive hair follicles, which are located on the chin, upper lip, and jawline, can respond more strongly, producing coarse hairs in these areas. Scalp follicles may shrink at this time, leading to volume loss and overall growth of shorter hairs. This is why taking systemic hormones in menopause may help — estrogen tempers the effects of the androgens.

4

Cognitive and Emotional Health in Menopause

Menopause doesn't just affect the body —
it can cause everything from brain fog to
irritability. It can even be associated with
mental health conditions like anxiety and
depression. This part covers the full spectrum
of how menopause can affect the mind and
offers information on how you can address
these issues if they occur.

DID YOU KNOW?

Often, long before menopause, women experience changes in their cognitive function. Forgetfulness, poor concentration, and brain fog can all happen in the years leading up to menopause, as hormone levels are changing. The good news is that these symptoms typically improve when all the hormonal swings are over.

Chapter **12**

Cognitive and Sensory Health

Fluctuating and declining estrogen levels can disrupt the parts of the brain that support memory, focus, sleep, and mood, bringing about symptoms like brain fog, poor word recall and concentration, and disrupted sleep. Estrogen also influences blood flow to the eyes and mouth. Menopausal women may experience changes like dry eyes or differences in taste or smell. This chapter covers how these cognitive and sensory symptoms arise, what effects they may have, and whether these symptoms typically improve over time.

Can Menopause Cause Memory Problems or Cognitive Changes?

Cognitive changes like lack of focus or difficulty identifying previously familiar faces can be seen in perimenopause. The hormonal shifts that occur in the years leading up to menopause, especially wildly fluctuating levels of estrogen, can cause memory lapses, brain fog, poor concentration, and difficulty finding words. Estrogen affects the hippocampus and the prefrontal cortex, the parts of the brain responsible for concentration and clear thinking. When estrogen levels fluctuate in perimenopause, there is a negative impact on these cognitive areas. These hormonal swings may also cause poor sleep, which can also have an impact on brain function. The good news is that, as the fluctuations lessen and menopause is reached, cognitive capabilities seem to stabilize and even sometimes improve.

Some of the effects on cognition and memory may also be related to nighttime flashes, causing a lack of good, deep sleep. When sleep is poor, this may (indirectly) worsen brain function, memory, and recall. Often, memory changes in menopause will improve with better sleep, stress management, and some "brain training" like learning a new language or regularly doing word puzzles.

Estrogen levels are connected to neurotransmitters (the chemical messengers present in the brain), like serotonin and dopamine. These neurotransmitters have an influence on focus, concentration, and cognitive processes. When estrogen levels fluctuate in perimenopause and decrease in menopause, the function of the neurotransmitters is compromised. This can result in brain fog, poor concentration, and memory issues.

The good news is that these symptoms are usually worst during the transition from perimenopause to menopause, when hormones are fluctuating. Women usually see improvements when the body adjusts to a new baseline in menopause. Also, lifestyle strategies like sleep hygiene, exercise, and stress management, as well as hormonal therapies, can greatly improve mental clarity and cognitive function.

What Can I Do to Improve Cognitive Function in Menopause?

The most effective intervention for improving brain function in perimenopause and menopause is to be sure to get regular, deep, and good-quality sleep. Most cognitive symptoms are amplified by poor sleep. Good sleep hygiene, treating any nighttime sweats or night flashes, assessing for sleep apnea, and possibly using a sleep aid or supplement can improve sleep.

When sleep improves, memory and focus often improve as well.

Exercise — both aerobic and resistance training — has been shown to improve cognitive function. Exercise supports brain health by increasing blood flow, decreasing inflammation, and elevating mood.

If there are underlying mental health issues, like anxiety or depression, making sure that these are managed appropriately with counseling, therapy, and possibly medications has been shown to ultimately improve cognitive function. Untreated depression can contribute to feelings of brain fog or lack of concentration.

Sugar and alcohol both have inflammatory effects on blood vessels, and ultimately brain function, especially with repeated exposure, so try to limit them as much as possible.

TIP

Mental engagement — social connections, reading, writing, language learning, and memory work — can all contribute to improvements in cognitive function.

What Is the Connection between Menopause and Dementia?

Although menopause is associated with some cognitive decline due to the decline in estrogen, dementia is another category altogether.

Dementia is a decline in cognitive function that is severe enough to interfere with a person's independence in everyday life. It's a clinical syndrome caused by various underlying conditions. In most cases, dementia is progressive and can't be explained solely by the normal aging process.

Although there is some anecdotal evidence that women who were placed on menopausal hormone therapy early in their menopausal transition may have less decline in their cognitive function, there are no studies that recommend using hormones, specifically estrogen, as a preventive treatment for dementia.

One type of dementia, called *vascular dementia,* occurs when blood vessels leading to the brain are blocked, inflamed, or stiff, not allowing adequate blood flow to the brain. Estrogen can have a positive impact on blood vessels, maintaining their elasticity and supporting blood flow. Starting on systemic estrogen while vessels are still healthy and supple may protect some regions of the brain associated with memory and recall (in the late perimenopause or early menopause years), but starting estrogen later (past age 65, or more than ten years into menopause) has not been shown to help cognition and may increase the risk of dementia.

Can Menopause Cause Changes in Vision and Eye Health?

Estrogen affects the production of tears from the tear ducts, and oil from the glands in the eyelids. Cataracts and glaucoma are more common with age, and a lack of estrogen can lead to dry eyes, blurry vision, or itching and burning.

The changes in vision and eye health may be partially impacted by decreasing estrogen levels, but many of the changes in vision and eye health are changes that are seen in aging itself. Dry eye syndrome is more common in menopausal women than in younger women. There may be a connection between lower estrogen levels and decreased tear production. Some women notice difficulty with night vision or an increase in light sensitivity. Aging and menopause also both increase the risk for cataracts.

Can Menopause Cause Changes in Taste and Smell?

The hormonal changes during perimenopause and menopause can cause changes in taste and smell, although these symptoms are less commonly discussed than other menopausal symptoms. Some menopausal women describe a sensation of burning in the mouth, with tingling or a scalded sensation on the gums, tongue, and lips without any visible lesions. Blood flow to the salivary glands may decrease, causing a sensation of dry mouth or a change in the way different foods taste. Sometimes familiar smells become unpleasant or less intense due to declining estrogen levels, which may change the way odors are perceived. Gum sensitivity and deficiency of certain vitamins can also cause changes in taste and smell.

Can Menopause Cause Changes in Hearing?

A decline in hearing is more likely to be caused by general aging than by menopause itself. Estrogen helps to keep blood vessels and nerves healthy, so there could be some changes with decreased blood flow to the nerves and blood vessels that assist in proper hearing. When estrogen levels fall, women may also develop sound sensitivity, but hearing loss is a part of aging for men and women alike.

What Kind of Neurological Symptoms Can Occur in Menopause?

Several neurological conditions and symptoms can be triggered in menopause. Headaches, migraines, new-onset dizziness, numbness and tingling, and restless leg syndrome are all conditions that may appear, recur, or flare in menopause. Estrogen influences nerve function and blood flow, so its decline can result in any of these neurological conditions worsening.

Your doctor should do a full evaluation to rule out other causes for these conditions, including nutritional deficiencies, infections, tumors, and autoimmune conditions. It is not recommended that estrogen be prescribed to treat any of these conditions. However, if a new set of symptoms occurs exactly at the time of declining hormones, menopause may be a contributor.

How Does Menopause Affect the Body's Circadian Rhythm?

The body's *circadian rhythm* (internal clock) regulates when we feel alert and when we feel sleepy. This internal system is influenced by estrogen and progesterone. When these hormones fluctuate in perimenopause and then decline in menopause, the sleep-wake cycle begins to change. It's common for menopausal women to experience difficulty falling asleep, staying asleep, or waking up much too early in the morning. Some *neurotransmitters* (brain chemicals) are responsible for having a calming effect. When levels of these transmitters (like GABA) are low in response to declining hormones, achieve restorative sleep becomes more difficult. Add to this the nighttime sweats that can also cause you to wake up, and menopause becomes a time of nightly sleep disruptions.

TIP

If sweating is the cause of your poor sleep, menopausal hormone therapy or other medical management may be warranted. Establishing sleep routines and focusing on restorative sleep can help restore healthy rhythms and reset that internal clock.

Chapter **13**

Mental and Emotional Health

enopause is a time of great change — not just because of the decline in estrogen, but because this is a time when many women see their children moving out of the house, their parents aging and needing more care, or their relationship with their significant other shifting. All these changes make women more vulnerable to anxiety and depression. Even if they aren't anxious or depressed, they're likely to be more irritable or stressed. This chapter explains the ways in which menopause affects mental and emotional health and offers strategies for tackling these issues and finding the support you need.

What Are the Best Ways to Manage Menopause-Related Anxiety?

Anxiety often becomes more intense or more noticeable during the transition to menopause. This is the time where estrogen and progesterone levels can start to fluctuate wildly, and will eventually decline to undetectable levels. These hormones play a role in regulating neurotransmitters like serotonin and dopamine, which affect anxiety and mood. Night sweats, which can disrupt sleep, can also cause increased anxiety, and physical symptoms like sweating and heart palpitations can occur, stimulating further feelings of anxiety and stress.

TIP

The most effective ways to treat menopausal anxiety is with a combination of therapies. Adhering to good sleep hygiene habits, taking part in regular exercise, practicing mindfulness and meditation, and limiting anything that seems to be a trigger for anxiety can be helpful. (Sometimes caffeine, alcohol, sugar, and stressful situations trigger anxiety symptoms.) Attending a support group or one-on-one therapy is helpful in many situations, especially cognitive behavioral therapy (CBT). If menopausal symptoms like hot flashes and night sweats seem to be triggering increased feelings of anxiety, treating these symptoms with hormone therapy can be helpful if you're a candidate. Medications specifically for treating anxiety or for anxiety and depression (such as sertraline, fluoxetine, venlafaxine, and desvenlafaxine) can be prescribed to reduce or relieve the feelings of anxiety. Some of these prescription medications have been found to also lessen vasomotor symptoms like hot flashes.

What Are the Best Ways to Manage Menopause-Related Depression?

Depression that has been present at certain key transition periods (adolescence, pregnancy, and postpartum) is likely to appear again or worsen at the time of the menopausal transition. Estrogen, which fluctuates in perimenopause and then declines, plays a key role in regulating the *neurotransmitters* (brain chemicals) responsible for regulating moods. When estrogen levels decline, mood stability is affected, which can trigger or worsen depression. Chronic sleep deprivation due to night sweats, sleep apnea, or other chronic conditions can also trigger or worsen depression, and life stressors can also play a role. Relationship issues, job changes, and family illness can trigger or worsen depression, contributing to feelings of helplessness or overwhelm.

A diagnosis of depression is made when experiencing certain ongoing key features like fatigue, low energy, changes in appetite or sleep, loss of interest in activities that were once enjoyable or stimulating, and a persistent feeling of sadness or low mood.

TIP

Treating depression during menopause should include a combination of things. Some type of therapy or counseling, especially CBT (which challenges negative thoughts and patterns), has been found to be the most effective treatment for depression in midlife and menopausal women. Other forms of therapy, like talk therapy or psychological counseling, can offer emotional support and tools to address stress, relationship issues, and general life stressors. Prescription medications for depression have been shown to be highly effective for women: They're often the first-line treatments for depression at any age. In menopause, if the symptoms of depression predated menopause or do not seem to be related to specific menopausal symptoms, anti-depressant medications can be very effective at relieving depressive symptoms and creating more stable moods.

If depression seems to be new in menopause and directly related to declining estrogen levels or paired with menopausal symptoms, sometimes a menopausal hormone therapy plan should be first-line treatment. Hormone therapy can often enhance the effect of prescription anti-depressant medications and can be combined if the situation warrants it.

Lifestyle changes should always be part of a menopausal plan to stay healthy and relieve depression. Regular exercise, consistent sleep, healthy nutrition, and stress management, along with social interactions and support, should form the basis of menopausal mood management.

What Are the Best Ways to Manage Menopause-Related Irritability?

Mood management in menopause can best be accomplished by identifying exactly what seems to be the cause of the irritability. The physical symptoms of menopause can seem disruptive to everyday life, and chronic discomfort can lead to increased irritability. If frequent hot flashes and night sweats are causing discomfort and irritability, you may find relief with hormones or nonhormonal treatments. If fatigue and joint or muscle pain are causing discomfort and irritability, a helpful exercise and stretching routine, getting enough sleep, or seeing a physical therapist may address these causes. If irritability seems to be exacerbating an underlying mental health condition like anxiety or depression, these issues should be addressed directly with therapy and possibly medications to treat these conditions. Sometimes limiting triggers (like caffeine and alcohol) can improve irritability, and focusing on a healthy lifestyle (regular exercise, proper nutrition) can go a long way toward lessening feelings of irritability, anxiety, and stress.

What Are the Best Ways to Manage Menopause-Related Mood Swings?

Mood swings are felt most acutely during *perimenopause*, the transition from reproductive years to menopausal years, which occurs mostly in the 40s (although it can occur as early as the late 30s). During perimenopause, the ovaries are still working, but not as efficiently or cyclically as they did when you were younger. The ovaries produce estrogen for much of the menstrual cycle and progesterone for about half the cycle, in response to ovulation. In perimenopause, these two hormones, estrogen and progesterone, are produced much more irregularly, causing variations in the amount of estrogen and/or progesterone present on any one day (sometimes in any given hour!). These variations or "swings" in hormone levels are thought to be most responsible for mood swings: During periods of time where both estrogen and/or progesterone are present, a feeling of well-being is more likely to be present. These are usually times of adequate energy and a sense of calm. When levels of these hormones plummet, it may be associated with brain fog, depression, anxiety, increased stress, and irritability. These fluctuations may happen irregularly, weekly, or daily, causing unstable feelings and mood swings.

Hormone stability is key to stabilizing these shifts. Hormonal stability can be achieved with combination hormonal contraception (certain types of estrogen and progesterone) for those who are candidates. A birth control pill, transdermal patch, or vaginal ring are all examples of hormonal treatments that work best to achieve stable levels of hormones for women who are not yet fully in menopause. They eliminate the hormonal swings, and with that, the mood swings and other symptoms that can be caused by fluctuating hormones.

Often when menopause is reached (12 full calendar months without a period), the hormonal fluctuations are gone because the ovaries are now making *no* estrogen and *no* progesterone. Mood swings often resolve at this time. If mood swings still appear to be present and bothersome in menopause, stability can be achieved with menopausal hormone therapy, which uses a much lower dose of estrogen and progesterone than contraceptives do. (Contraceptives aim to *suppress* ovarian function to prevent pregnancy, whereas menopausal hormone therapy aims to relieve symptoms.)

What Are Some Effective Ways to Manage Stress during Menopause?

Usually a combined approach to managing stress is most effective. Lifestyle approaches like getting enough sleep, eating healthy foods, and getting regular exercise are helpful at any age, but in menopause, these habits are essential.

Techniques like mindfulness and meditation have been shown to reduce both hot flashes and anxiety. Support groups, as well as support from family and friends, can be helpful in decreasing the stress of menopause. The right mix of treatments depends on symptoms, health conditions, and preferences.

TIP

Meditation, deep breathing exercises, and CBT are some ways to manage stress. Numerous apps are focused on meditation; examples include Headspace and Insight Timer. Similarly, you can find numerous books and websites devoted to breathing exercises; *Breathing Exercises For Dummies* by Shamash Alidina (Wiley) is one example. Most therapists, whether in-person or online, are familiar with CBT. There are also medications that directly treat anxiety and chronic stress situations in combination with lifestyle changes and therapy.

What Are the Benefits of Cognitive Behavioral Therapy for Menopausal Symptoms?

CBT is a structured, evidence-based form of talk therapy that can help people identify and change patterns in their thoughts, emotions, and behaviors. It's one of the most effective types of psychotherapy. CBT has been found to help with vasomotor symptoms like hot flashes and night sweats. It's also helpful for chronic pain, and it's one of the most effective treatments for insomnia. Sessions are usually weekly for a determined period of time and focus on setting goals, identifying problems, and replacing problematic thoughts with more realistic ones.

TIP

CBT-i Coach (https://mobile.va.gov/app/cbt-i-coach) is a mobile app developed by the U.S. Department of Veterans Affairs designed to support CBT for insomnia. Apps like Seren or Evia may be helpful for vasomotor symptoms in menopause.

Are There Support Groups for Women Going through Menopause?

You can find groups of women sharing the experience of menopause online and in person.

In a private Facebook Community called Menopause Chicks, women discuss symptoms, wellness tips, and treatments. On Reddit at www.reddit.com/r/Menopause/, they discuss symptoms, hormones, and treatments. There is also an online community called Red Hot Mamas (https://redhotmamas.org), which offers education and support for women going through menopause.

Menopause can be a frustrating experience, but you're not alone, and you can find other women going through the same things you are.

Index

A

Academy of Nutrition and Dietetics, 34

Active Menopause Life website, 35

acupuncture, 38–39

adrenal health, menopause impacts, 65–67

age of menopause, 6

aging, 13, 87, 98, 108

androgens (male hormones), 58, 79, 92, 98, 99

anxiety, 13, 106
  treatment of, 114–115

appetite, menopause impacts, 64

aromatherapy, 40–41

asthma, 76, 77

autoimmune diseases, 80

B

balance problems, 83–84

basal metabolic rate, 62

birth control pills

side effects during menopause, 22–23

therapeutic uses, 22

black cohosh herb, 43–44

blood sugar levels, 62–63, 65

body odor changes, 79–80

body temperature regulation, 10–11

bone health, menopause impacts
  bone resorption rate, 85
  bone supplements, 89
  joint pain and stiffness, 86
  muscle mass and strength, 86–88

bone-regulating hormones, menopause impacts, 68

bone supplements, 89

brain training, 104

breast cancer patient, menopausal hormone therapy, 25–26

C

calcium supplement, 89

cancer risk
cervical cancers, 59–60, 74
hormone-sensitive cancer, 74
risk factors, 74

cardiovascular exercise, 35

cardiovascular health, menopause impacts
lower estrogen levels, 70
preventive maintenance, 70–71

cervical cancers, 59–60, 74

chiropractic care, 42–43

cholesterol profile, menopause impacts, 67–68, 71–72

circadian rhythm (internal clock), menopause impacts, 110–111

cognitive and memory changes
dementia, 106–107
in hearing, 109
to improve cognitive function, 105–106
lifestyle strategies, 105
nighttime flashes, 104

taste and smell, 108–109
vision and eye health, 108

cognitive behavioral therapy (CBT), 120–121

comfort foods, 64

contraindicated women for hormone therapy
breast cancer history, 19–20
deep vein thrombosis, 20
heart attack, 20
high blood pressure, 20
stroke, 20
unexpected bleeding, 20

cortisol levels, 65, 66

creatine, 88

D

dehydroepiandrosterone (DHEA), 54, 58, 66

dementia, 106–107
vascular dementia, 107

depression, 13, 106
diagnosis of, 115–116
lifestyle modifications, 116–117
treatment of, 116

diabetes, 63–64

diet, 70

Dietary Approaches to Stop Hypertension (DASH), 32

Mediterranean diet, 32

plant-based diet, 32

restrictions, 34

Dietary Approaches to Stop Hypertension (DASH), 32

don quai herb, 44

dry eye syndrome, 108

E

education and support for women, 121

elinzanetant, 24

endocrine health, menopause impacts

on blood glucose levels, 65

cholesterol profile, changes in, 67–68

on cortisol levels, 65, 66

on dehydroepiandrosterone (DHEA) levels, 66

on thyroid hormone levels, 65, 66

endorphins, 34–35

endothelium, 72

esophageal sphincter, 75

estrogen, 10–12, 41, 48, 54, 56–58, 62, 64, 68, 75, 77, 80, 114

in blood sugar levels, 63

in blood vessels, 72, 78

in bone health, 85–86

cardioprotective effects, 71

in cardiovascular health, 70

cognitive and memory changes, 104–105

for dementia treatment, 107

dosage forms, 18, 55

in hair growth phase, 92, 98

in hearing, 109

in muscle mass and strength, 86–88

in musculoskeletal health, 82–83

in nail health, 96–97

in neurotransmitters regulation, 115

prescribing rules, 18

protective effect on kidneys, 78

silicone ring, 54–56

in skin hydration, 92

estrogen *(continued)*

in skin pigmentation, 94–95

suppository/vaginal estrogen pill, 54, 55

thyroid hormone levels, 65

topical estrogen, 54, 59

vaginal estrogen creams, 54, 55

in vision and eye health, 108

exercises, 34–35, 70, 106

F

fatigue, 81–82

fezolinetant, 24

Food and Drug Administration (FDA), 44

G

gabapentin, 24–25

gastroesophageal reflux disease (GERD), 75

gastrointestinal health, menopause impacts, 75–76

genital tissues, hormones impact, 55–56

Global Statement on Testosterone Therapy, 51

gum sensitivity and deficiency, 109

H

hair growth

anagen phase/growth phase, 92

androgen hormone, 98, 99

estrogen hormone, 98, 99

hair loss management, 95–96

lifestyle strategies, 97–98

prescription medications, 93

telogen phase/shedding phase, 92

hair loss management, 95–96

hearing loss, 109

herbal remedies, 43–44

high-density lipoprotein (HDL) cholesterol, 67

hormonal stability, 118–119

hormone-sensitive cancer, 74

hot flashes, 8–10

cardiovascular disease, 71

estrogen, regulation with, 12

herbal remedies for,
43, 44

medications, 24–25

human papilloma virus
(HPV), 59, 60, 74

hypothalamus, 11, 12

hysterectomy, 26

I

immune system,
menopause impacts,
80–81

irritable bladder
symptoms, 12

J

joint pain and stiffness, 86

K

Kava herb, 44

kidney health, menopause
impacts, 78

L

libido
declining, 50
definition, 49
enhancement, 50–52
responsive libido,
49–50

lifestyle modifications
benefits of, 30–31
for cognitive and memory
changes, 105
for depression, 116–117
dietary changes,
31–32, 34
exercises, 34–35
for hair growth, 97–98
for nail health, 98
nutritional counseling,
33–34
for skin, 97–98
weight management, 36

liver health, menopause
impacts, 77–78

long-term health
implications of
menopause, 8

low-density lipoprotein
(LDL) cholesterol,
67, 70

lung disease, 77

M

massage therapy, 41–42

medical consultation, 7–8

medications for hot flashes
elinzanetant, 24
fezolinetant, 24

medications for hot flashes
  (continued)
 gabapentin, 24–25
 oxybutynin, 25
 paroxetine, 25
meditation, benefits of, 38
Mediterranean diet, 32
menopausal hormone
  therapy, 96, 98, 107, 111
 in breast cancer patient,
  25–26
 contraindicated women,
  19–21
 estrogen, 10–12, 18–19
 in ovarian/endometrial
  cancer patient, 26–27
 progesterone, 18, 19
 risks and benefits, 21
 testosterone, 19, 23–24
menopause. *See also*
  specific entries
 age of, 6
 definition of, 5–6, 21, 57
Menopause Chicks
  website, 121
metabolic health,
  menopause impacts
 appetite changes, 64
 basal metabolic rate, 62
 blood sugar levels,
  62–63, 65

diabetes, 63–64
low-density lipoprotein
  (LDL) cholesterol
  level, 62
mindfulness techniques, 38
mobility exercises, 35
mood management, 117
mood swings, 118–119
muscle health
 mass and strength, 86–88
 protein supplementation,
  88
musculoskeletal health,
  menopause impacts,
  82–83

N

nail health, 96–97
 lifestyle strategies, 98
neurological symptoms,
  109–110
neurotransmitters,
  110, 115
night sweats, 8, 10,
  11, 114
 estrogen, regulation
  with, 12
 herbal remedies for, 44
nighttime flashes, 104
nutritional counseling,
  33–34

O

obstructive sleep apnea, 77

oophorectomy, 26

oral finasteride, 96

oral health, menopause impacts, 78–79

osteopenia, 86

osteoporosis, 68, 83, 86

ovarian/endometrial cancer patient, menopausal hormone therapy, 26–27

ovulation, 6, 56

oxybutynin, 25

P

pap test, 59–60

paroxetine, 25

perimenopause, 6, 57, 81, 104, 105, 108, 110, 115

mood swings, 118–119

phytoestrogens, 43

plant-based diet, 32

prediabetes, 63, 64

progesterone, 18, 19, 64, 75, 77, 80, 114

progestin, 18

psychological effects, 13–14

R

rapid eye movement (REM) sleep, 8

Reddit website, 121

Red Hot Mamas online community, 121

reproductive health, menopause impacts

on reproductive cycles, 57

to reproductive hormones, 57–58

to reproductive organs, 56

reproductive hormones, 57–58

resistance exercises, 35

respiratory health, menopause impacts, 76–77

responsive libido, 49–50

restorative sleep, 111

S

sexual health

affecting factors, 48–49

intimacy changes, 48

libido changes, 49–52

shortness of breath, 77

silicone ring, 54–56

skin impacts
  dark spots/redness, 92
  dryness/itching, 91
  hyperpigmentation (dark spots), 95
  hypopigmentation (white spots), 95
  lifestyle strategies, 97–98
  moisturizers, 92
  skin care routine, 93–94
  skin pigmentation, 94–95
skin pigmentation, 94–95
sleep disturbances, 11
  estrogen, regulation with, 12, 115
  irritable bladder symptoms, 12
sleep hygiene, 82
stress, 65, 76, 82
  management of, 119–120
symptoms of menopause
  common symptoms, 6
  duration, 7
  hot flashes (see hot flashes)
  medical consultation, 7–8
  new-onset psychological symptoms, 13
  night sweats (see night sweats)

severity of, 7
vaginal dryness (see vaginal dryness)

T
testosterone, 19, 23–24, 51, 58
  positive impact, 23
  side effects of, 24
thyroid health, menopause impacts, 65, 66
topical estrogen, 54, 59
topical minoxidil, 96

U
urinary health, menopause impact, 58–59

V
vaginal dryness, 7, 8, 26, 27, 47
  causes of, 52
  dehydroepiandrosterone (DHEA), 54
  local hormone therapy, 54
  lubricants, 53
  moisturizers, 53–54
  oral medications, 54
  topical estrogen, 54
  treatment, 48–49, 52–54

vaginal estrogen creams, 54, 55

vaginal estrogen pill/ suppository, 54, 55

vascular dementia, 107

vision and eye health, 108

vitamin D, 68, 89

W

weight-bearing activity, 35

weight gain, 35–36

  management, 36

Y

yoga

  apps and channels, 40

  benefits, 39

  for relaxation and sleep, 39

  for strength and balance, 39

About the Author

Rebecca Levy-Gantt, DO, is a board-certified obstetrician and gynecologist and a Nationally Certified Menopause Practitioner whose areas of expertise include menopause, perimenopause, and hormonal management. She has had her own OB-GYN private practice for the past 11 years and has more than 30 years of experience in women's health. She spent the first half of her medical career in New York, and for the last 15 years has worked in Napa, California. Dr. Levy-Gantt is the author of two memoirs — *Womb With A View* and *Motherhood, Medicine & Me* (both published by Wordrunner Press) — and *Perimenopause For Dummies* (published by Wiley). She is currently in the process of retiring from clinical practice to focus on teaching and consulting. Dr. Levy-Gantt's interests include traveling, learning languages, reading, and spending time with her husband, Bill, and their five children and four grandchildren.

Dedication

This book is dedicated to my daughter Danielle, who has always been my champion and has supported me throughout the writing process. Danielle embodies intelligence, humor, and fearless independence. She's a hilarious, sex-positive force of nature and will one day be a kick-ass menopausal woman. All my love.

Publisher's Acknowledgments

Senior Managing Editor:
Kristie Pyles

Executive Editor:
Tracy Boggier

Editor: Elizabeth Kuball

Production Editor:
Magesh Elangovan

**Cover Design and
Image:** Wiley

Special Help:
Carmen Krikorian